EQUITY

&

HEALTH

Views from the
Pan American
Sanitary Bureau

Pan American Health Organization
Regional Office of the
World Health Organization
525 23rd Street, N.W.
Washington, D.C. 20037 U.S.A.

PAHO Library Cataloguing in Publication Data

Pan American Health Organization
    Equity and Health: Views from the Pan American Sanitary Bureau
Washington, D.C: PAHO, © 2001.- (Occasional Publication No. 8)

ISBN 92 75 12288 1

1. Title   II. Series

1. EQUITY IN HEALTH CONDITIONS
2. POVERTY
3. SOCIOECONOMIC FACTORS
4. HEALTH FINANCING
5. HEALTH STATUS INDICATORS
6. AMERICAS

LC HC79.P187e 2001

TABLE OF CONTENTS

PART 3.   MAKING HEALTH EQUITY WORK AT THE COUNTRY LEVEL

PREFACE

Over the last several years, the concept of equity has emerged as a primary guiding principle for the work of the Pan American Health Organization (PAHO). In particular, PAHO has been gathering information on, and examining issues related to, disparities in health in the Americas, especially as they relate to socioeconomic factors. Research findings from this effort have important implications for the Organization's work, in that they provide an empirical basis on which to build claims of health inequities and move toward a more equitable distribution of the determinants of health outcomes. The development of a robust interpretation of the concept of equity is crucial for the advancement of its application in the provision of appropriate technical cooperation by the Organization. The articles gathered in this publication represent an important step in that direction, in the measure in which they represent the status of the issues and dilemmas faced by the PAHO Secretariat in making equity an operational concept for its work in the Region. The challenge immediately before the authors is to show how this principle and the insights it yields into the distribution of health—dependent as this is on differences in education, income, class, ethnicity and race, geographic location, gender, and other distinctions—can underpin the Organization's work at the operational level and be incorporated into technical cooperation activities.

George A. O. Alleyne
Director

INTRODUCTION

In October 1999, PAHO held its first Organization-wide technical discussion of equity, sharing perspectives developed by different Organizational divisions and among those working at the country level. This publication includes the presentations made at that meeting and is intended to provide a broad basis for discussion as well as to stimulate future thought. The collection stands as an initial effort to interpret the concept of equity for application to the various areas of PAHO's work.

The individual articles were developed independently and reflect different approaches to the interpretation of health equity. Many of the perspectives expressed in the collection extend from the conceptual work developed by other scholars and researchers or emerge from PAHO's ongoing work with collaborating institutions. Present project partners include the Rockefeller Foundation, the World Bank, UNDP, and CARICOM, as well as several universities and professional and academic associations in the Region. This diversity has presented challenges of its own. The job of the editors has been to clarify the authors' ideas and otherwise encourage dialogue that will eventually result in conclusions, recommendations, and actions to be taken. A common understanding of how to translate the concept would allow us to apply it to PAHO's programs and technical cooperation, and to identify concrete and practical interventions and establish priorities which will contribute to increased equity in health in the countries of the Americas.

This collection is organized into three sections: "Conceptual and Contextual Aspects of Health Equity," "Priorities for Incorporating Equity into Technical Cooperation in Health," and "Making Health Equity Work at the Country Level."

In the introductory chapter, Sir George Alleyne, the Director of PAHO, provides a context for discussing equity and health, including the philosophical tenets of the concept and its recent historical development within the international health arena. In particular, he emphasizes the contribution of the "Black Report" and the "Acheson Report," especially in their emphasis on social determinants of health. Further, Dr. Alleyne links past concerns with poverty to current equity and health projects, noting that current research indicates that not only absolute levels of poverty but also relative deprivation appears to affect health disparities. Finally, Dr. Alleyne provides suggestions for the role that organizations such as PAHO and WHO can play in promoting equitable health situations, focusing on information collection and technical cooperation.

In "Assessing Equity in Health: Conceptual Criteria," Bambas and Casas build and expand on the definition of equity for health developed by Margaret Whitehead. They explore the implications of Whitehead's criteria for establishing health disparities as equitable or inequitable, including avoidability and choice, but also including a much overlooked criterion of responsible agency. The discussion provides a more detailed explication of each of the criteria and explains why they are relevant to the issue, demonstrating how they can then be applied to specific situations in order to gauge the level of equity or inequity present. This model provides a basis on which subsequent discussions of equity that present empirical information on disparities among populations can be guided and interpreted.

The second chapter, "Health Disparities in Latin America and the Caribbean: The Role of Social and Economic Determinants," by Casas, Dachs, and Bambas, provides an overview of the current empirical information available on various aspects of socioeconomic inequalities in the Region. The authors first establish the general social and economic context of Latin America and the Caribbean, including changes in the distribution of income and education, both within and between countries and regions. After discussing the present paucity of information in the Region, the article reviews the data available for distributions of health between countries, and focuses on disparities within countries: among groups with different levels of income and education, populations living in different geographic locations, among ethnic groups, between men and women, among those with different levels of physical and financial access to health services, and for migrants. Finally, strategic areas for the Organization are suggested, as are conclusions and issues for further investigation.

The next two articles examine how to craft policies to promote equity in health. Using the concept of "developmental cocktails" to create intersectoral synergy, Eduardo Doryan raises key issues in combining an equity approach with attention to poverty to create policy that accelerates the pace of human development in underdeveloped countries. The question, as he poses it, is how to invest resources to simultaneously create growth and decrease inequality. Doryan then ties the discussion into the three core issues of the upcoming *World Development Report*—empowerment of the disadvantaged; security, livelihood, and risk management policies for nations; and opportunity for investment and sustainable economic development. These core issues, he says, can be used as a cross-sectoral framework for human development.

Adam Wagstaff demonstrates how to use empirical findings to link research to policymaking in order to further two of the broad goals of the health sector: 1) income protection, specifically out-of-pocket payments and income loss due to illness and 2) focusing on the health of the poor through access to health care and the non-medical determinants of health. Intercountry comparisons show how the architecture of systems creates differential financial burdens between income groups through regressivity of payments, threat of poverty due to out of pocket payments, and the availability of private insurance vs. publicly funded systems. Wagstaff then provides a methodology for predicting the health impact of specific interventions, such as reducing travel time for the poor to medical facilities, broadening insurance coverage, and improving the quality of medical services.

Framing the discussion within social, economic, and cultural human rights and modern concepts of social justice, Piedad Córdova makes a cogent argument that the State is the responsible agent for ensuring fair background conditions and institutions as well as addressing those social factors that affect health equity. Córdova emphasizes how factors that especially affect women and ethnic minorities, such as violence, exclusion, marginalization, and discrimination, generate inequitable social conditions that can eventually manifest as health inequities. The State has the duty to recognize social factors of inequity and progressively address them and create fair background institutions in which the population can direct political will. Further, the egalitarian construction of political power; reduction of corruption; and support for economic, social, and cultural rights can increase resources available for the equitable construction of a society. Córdova suggests that, based on this discussion and the need to strengthen social institutions and political processes, international cooperation should focus on information gathering and dissemination, and training, so that countries may attain the capacity to make their own development plans.

The book's second section focuses on equity in relation to several priority areas for the Organization, including establishing measuring methodologies as well as addressing 1) risk factors in disease prevention and control, 2) maternal mortality, 3) safe drinking water, and 4) access to and financing of health services. These articles present current information from LAC on the issue, including statistics and measuring practices, as well as methodological problems and additional information needed in order to establish equity in health.

"La Medición de las Desigualdades en Salud" ("The Measurement of Health Inequalities") discusses the use of several indicators of health disparities, as well as the purposes of and complications involved in using them. Measurement indicators of inequality can help to determine when there is equity in health, and how to identify equity gaps. The authors discuss relative and absolute measures of inequality, population attributable risk, the slope index of inequality and relative index of inequality, and the Gini coefficient and concentration index. The article also explains the problems of taking into account only extremes of privilege and deprivation, and concludes by emphasizing that measuring and documenting inequalities is imperative for establishing a basis on which to develop policies and interventions.

The next chapter, "Noncommunicable Diseases and Risk Factor Surveillance," deals with how to address equity concerns in the area of risk factors for noncommunicable diseases, which tend to be linked to both behavior and biology, two factors with seemingly different implications in terms of *avoidability* and *choice*. For instance, behaviors are usually thought of as chosen, but the concentration of risky behaviors among those in lower socioeconomic groups raises questions as to the degree of choice actually at work within this population group. As our perceptions of choice change, so do specific senses of avoidability, e.g. behaviors are avoidable in a different sense if they are based on sociological/cultural phenomena such as advertising rather than individual autonomous choice. Other risk factors for disease, such as exposure to health hazards, also are discussed, as are limitations of the measurements, quality of registries, and the difficulties of mixing data sources. The authors provide suggestions for reducing inequalities and give an example of how to use information on the prevalence of risk factors among socioeconomic groups to guide program planning.

In the area of health promotion and protection, maternal mortality is strongly concentrated among those women in low socioeconomic positions. Because maternal mortality has a significant impact on the affected women and their families and is also highly avoidable, addressing this health problem presents great potential for reducing one area of health inequity. "Health Equity and Maternal Mortality" provides a brief overview of the magnitude and causes of maternal mortality, the context of delivery practices in the Region, and the causes of insufficient attendant care at birth. The authors then review typical measures of maternal mortality, including maternal mortality ratio and rate, as well as lifetime risk. The discussion then turns to limitations of the measures and difficulties with surveillance before reviewing some of the disparities in health expectancies, including maternal mortality, for different socioeconomic and geographical groups. The authors conclude with recommendations for action to reduce maternal mortality, as well as an argument for why the topic is a priority area for health equity.

"Health Equity in Relation to Safe Drinking Water Supply" focuses on access to safe drinking water and demonstrates the potential health impact and high stratification of access according to geographic location and income. While the health equity argument turns on the basic need of all people for safe drinking water, the authors expand their discussion to include the necessity of broad population access to quality water for economic development. Because many governmental sectors as well as subpopulations have an interest in broad population access to quality water, the health sector must act in tandem with other sectors to advocate for infrastructure development.

The next chapter, "Access to and Financing of Health Care," addresses how to assess equity in access to and financing of personal health care services. The chapter provides some empirical information on disparities in access to health care services and the differential burdens of financing among subpopulations in the Region. The authors also address measurement and surveillance issues related to access to services and the financial burdens of access, and discuss geographical, economic, and cultural barriers to access. The discussion concludes with a proposal to reduce such inequalities.

In the publication's third section, several authors comment on their national-level perspectives of equity and health. Richard Van West-Charles ties equity to human development by drawing in concepts of deprivation and vulnerability as key factors. He contends that although health systems generally focus on curative medicine to address population health needs, the medical model is not a sufficient paradigm for the health system. Further, technology should benefit all segments of the population, and equity analyses should take into account both public and private sector resources. Van West-Charles ends his remarks with comments on financing and consumer choice, three facets of access to care, and the complimentarity of efficiency/effectiveness and equity.

Hernán Málaga describes the relationships between material living conditions and the health status of populations in both Venezuela and Colombia, as well as the potential benefit of the healthy communities strategy in the effort to decrease inequalities and inequities. He provides specific examples of interventions developed in Colombia to address health problems declared as important by the communities themselves, and notes the basic principles that are guiding the country's health sector reforms. This analysis of the situation leads him to the formulation of eleven guidelines for technical cooperation in health in Colombia.

Finkelman provides a framework of reference for Brazil by analyzing the Constitution and the consequent legal instruments related to health, as well as the main aspects of health sector reforms and the health care system organization, as they relate to equity. He then relates this frame of reference to the deep inequalities in Brazilian society, and presents evidence of these inequalities in material living conditions, health status, resources and coverage of health care services, and the financing of health care. By confronting the reality of inequality with the existing legal framework, he suggests a set of possible guidelines for technical cooperation in health in Brazil to address the problem of inequity.

"Agua para todos en el país de la fantasia" is a fable on the modernization of the State, the privatization of water services in developing countries, and the consequences for vulnerable populations in these countries. In this chapter, Paúlo César Pinto describes a possible scenario of what might happen in this process for both the economically better-off (i.e. improvements—with higher costs) as well as for the poor (an even smaller likelihood of access to quality water services in the near future). He ends by posing nine questions to be answered in relation to how to expand the provision of safe water to economically depressed areas and population groups.

Finally, Fernando Lolas expounds on the necessity of good theory for practical action in "Ethics, Equity, and Practices in Health Institutions." Theory "unmasks reality" and shows the infinite variety of circumstances, thereby strengthening our ability to transform values into policy and action. And while theory requires time for reflection, the urgency of work for those in the health field can create barriers for the integration of theory and practice. After an explication of the general usefulness of ethical theory to practical action, Lolas addresses the role of social institutions as conduits of justice, because, as he says, they convert ideals into practical principles and ideas into action.

Although equity in health has begun to flow freely into the mainstream literature, there is much work left to be done. "The Black Report" and the "Acheson Report" as well as the work of Margaret Whitehead, which were developed for the context of the United Kingdom, remain seminal conceptual and operational documents. But the concepts, values, and assumptions of these documents should be tested against the cultural context of other countries, which have different organizational and technical abilities and levels of development.

The articles presented here do not pretend to be the last word on the subject of equity and health in the Region of the Americas, but are meant to bring awareness to those working in different areas of health equity of each other's work and perspectives. PAHO expects that as the topic continues to develop, communication and sharing knowledge on the topic will become a main priority for health equity in its own right. To this end, PAHO, through the Division of Health and Human Development, in association with the International Society for Health Equity, has established an equity email listserv that regularly distributes documents, news, and other relevant information on the development of this emerging and rapidly growing field of research and advocacy. We welcome comments on the perspectives presented in this publication, which can be sent to *HDP@paho.org*.

The Editors

PART 1

CONCEPTUAL AND CONTEXTUAL ASPECTS OF HEALTH EQUITY IN THE AMERICAS

EQUITY AND HEALTH

George A. O. Alleyne[1, 2]

According to Aristotle's Eudemian Ethics, the following quotation was inscribed over the temple of Lelo at Delos: "Justice is fairest and Health is best. But to win one's desire is the pleasantest."

I have always been inspired by this and have come to believe that the practice of medicine, especially that related to the medicine of groups of people, provides the ideal opportunity to combine the concerns about health and justice and win one's desire. Just about the time I joined the Pan American Health Organization (PAHO) nineteen years ago, my interest in the relation between justice and health was stimulated further by a small book written by Alastair Campbell, from the Department of Ethics of the University of Edinburgh, entitled *Medicine, Health and Justice*.

Campbell dealt with the issue of ethics and priorities in medicine and stressed the value of individual freedom and needs. If patients were consumers and health care workers were providers, then there was a possibility that injustice could be committed if health care was relegated to being an ordinary commodity that was exchanged between providers and consumers in the market place. Equity for him was a matter of distributive justice, and those with the same needs or capacities should be treated equally. Of course, it was difficult to find adequate standards

for needs. But the part that struck me most forcibly was his treatment of justice as fairness in relation to health in the context of a "balance of freedom, equality and fraternity."

He went on to describe John Rawls' Theory of Justice as it bore on health, referring to the social contract theory of justice in which the "Original Position" is derived by rational individuals devising a society under "a veil of ignorance." The two basic principles that Rawls formulated are that each person should have rights to maximum liberty compatible with a similar system of liberty for all and that inequalities are to be arranged so that they benefit maximally the least advantaged. These basic liberties were described as the "equal liberties of citizenship" which must be tempered by equality in a good society. I have always wondered why these liberties or basic values did not include specifically, as appears in several other declarations on rights and liberties, the right or liberty to have access to those measures necessary to ensure health.

Health must be one of the ends or states that society will pursue. Health, however produced, is an essential aspect of human development, and I will resist any disciplinary arrogance that would induce me to claim that it is the best. However, health, as is material wealth, is important for enhancing the possibility a human being has to flourish and enjoy life's options. Without it, human beings are limited in the life paths that can be followed. If one believes that it is intrinsic to our condi-

[1] Director, Pan American Health Organization.
[2] Adapted from a presentation originally made at the XI World Congress of Psychiatry on "Psychiatry on New Thresholds," Hamburg, Germany, 6–11 August 1999.

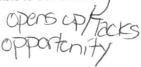
opens up/lacks opportunity

tion that we have the same life chances, then one may conclude that it is morally correct to seek health equality as far as possible.

I have emphasized repeatedly in PAHO that the two basic value principles that should guide our work and our technical cooperation are the search for equity in health and a Pan American approach that sees the countries of the Americas joining hands in the kinds of enterprises that lead to Health For All. I am not alone in this, as the European Region of the World Health Organization (WHO) has placed Equity in Health as the second of thirty-eight targets within its new Policy for Health for All. The target is described thus: "By the year 2020, the health gap between socioeconomic groups within countries should be reduced by at least one-fourth in all Member States, by substantially improving the level of health of disadvantaged groups."

In its first policy, published in 1985, equity was accorded the first place among the targets, and I must recognize the sterling work of persons like Margaret Whitehead ensuring that equity is a point of major interest in this Region.

We are not original in this concern, as the issue of equity in health and in other areas of human experience has been the subject of debate by philosophers for many years; more recently, economists have bent their minds to unraveling some of its implications and making proposals to measure and perhaps achieve such equity. As Director of PAHO, and being neither a philosopher nor an economist, it has not been an easy task to try to grasp the essentials of the two sets of propositions—that is, those of the philosophers and the economists—and at the same time devise some practical applications for an organization that is committed to cooperating with countries that have a wide range of social, economic, and health conditions, but are all united in the belief that human action can improve the health of all, particularly the disadvantaged.

The issue for me is not only equity in health outcomes, but also equity in the various determinants of health. There is wide acceptance of the view that equity refers to differences that are unnecessary or reducible and are unfair and unjust. The concept of fairness obviously involves a moral judgment and is, therefore, intrinsically difficult. As is the case with health outcomes, the inequities in health determinants are those that should not exist. Every person should, in terms of equity, have the opportunity to access those sanitary and social measures necessary to protect, promote, and maintain or recover health.

Because of biological constraints, there are differences or inequalities in health outcomes or health status that are unavoidable or irreducible. By the same token, there are myriad examples of differences or inequalities in health outcomes that are unnecessary and, therefore, represent inequities. There are differences between rural and urban areas and between ethnic groups, differences on the basis of gender, intergenerational differences, and, the most marked of all, are the differences between rich and poor both between and within countries. One of the starkest and most egregious examples of unjust differences in our Region is with regard to maternal mortality. A pregnant woman in the poorest country of our hemisphere has about a fifty times greater risk of dying as a result of her pregnancy than a woman in the rich countries. This may be related to the fact that whereas almost all women in the rich countries are attended by a trained attendant during childbirth, this happens in just about 50% of the time in the poorest countries. To take another example, the population attributable risk for dying from acute respiratory infections was calculated to show that if all countries had the same mortality rate for children under 5 years old as does North America, there would be 93% fewer deaths from these infections in this age group in Latin America and the Caribbean.

Although almost every country in the world has data showing the differences in health outcomes, I refer frequently to the United Kingdom where there is a tradition of more than 150 years of collecting and analyzing health data. The famous Black Report of 1980

records are important

was a seminal work on the inequalities in health and the policies necessary to promote and restore health. Even though the report caused little positive domestic reaction at the time, it was and continues to be the stimulus for debate and research in the international arena on the inequalities of health outcome and the means to address them.

More recently another study on inequalities in health in the UK has been conducted, and the findings have been published in what is known as the Acheson Report, after the chairman, Sir Donald Acheson. The report documents the persisting inequalities in health and states, "... for many measures of health, inequalities have either remained the same or have widened in recent decades." This still comes as a surprise to many of us who had imagined that universal access to health care services, as obtains in the National Health Service, would have served to decrease the inequalities as the overall mortality continued to fall. The report "adopts the socioeconomic model of health and its inequalities" and posits that the capacity of the personal behavior and lifestyles of individuals to affect health is significantly modulated by the social and community influences in which a given individual operates. In addition, there is a wide range of living and working conditions that can positively or negatively affect the health outcomes, and the health care services are included among these conditioning factors, but are not given any primacy in affecting outcome.

The data clearly show the impact of social class on health. In spite of criticisms of the formulation of the social classes, there is now overwhelming evidence of the influence of social hierarchy on health. In the classic work *Why Some People Are Healthy and Others Not* by Evans and his colleagues, Renaud makes a most definitive statement:

> The lower one is situated in the social hierarchy as defined by work, lodging, education, income or whatever; the lower one's probability of staying in good health and the lower one's life expectancy. This is the most frequent

and most pervasive of all the observations made in the history of public health.

The fact that health outcomes are to a large measure socially determined gives hope that these social conditions, if altered, can lead to improved health. The Acheson Report notes that in order to reduce health inequalities, "further steps should be taken to reduce income inequalities and improve the living standards of poor households." This recommendation is remarkably accurate in that it addresses both the aspect of difference in income and the absolute level of income that is associated with poverty. There has often been debate as to whether it is income distribution or poverty that has the major impact on health. The answer is that the predominance of one or other depends very much on the economic status of the population examined.

The relation of poverty to ill health has been known for centuries, and the classic work of medical historians such as Sigerist outlines the evolution of that relationship. He describes the major lines of thought of the eighteenth century when activists like Johann Peter Frank recognized poverty as a major cause of disease and advocated for a police function in public health. The industrial revolution accentuated the appalling health living conditions of the poor and led to the utilitarian approaches of reformers like Chadwick towards improving the health of the poor in the nineteenth century.

It is appropriate here to point out the role of one of my medical heroes, Rudolf Virchow, whose leadership of the health reform movement in this country has left a remarkable legacy in terms of social security that includes health benefits. It was about 150 years ago that he investigated an outbreak of relapsing fever in Silesia and came to the conclusion that the causes were essentially social. According to Sigerist, he recommended prosperity, education, and liberty, which can develop only on the basis of complete and unrestricted democracy.

The impact of poverty on health is still evident today, and in every country it will be the poor who are the most disadvantaged, both in terms of health outcomes and in access to the factors that make for good health. Poverty is associated with mental as well as physical illness, and there are good data to show that low socioeconomic status is associated with higher rates of psychopathology. But as the Report on World Mental Health points out, "although poverty is linked to mental ill health, economic prosperity does not translate directly into either personal or social well-being."

An analysis by Kawachi and his colleagues describes lucidly the two approaches to the economic situations associated with ill health. There is the focus on absolute poverty, with the need that is expressed so often today of eliminating or eradicating poverty. These expressions borrow from the image of disease control and eradication but, although attractive as slogans, are not usually useful in operational terms. The other focus is on relative deprivation, where it is the difference in income between groups perhaps at any level of wealth that is a major determinant of health outcome. It is important to make this differential. Poverty affects the individual's capacity to maintain or recover his or her health and in addition impacts on the societal environment that itself will affect health. Relative deprivation or, in its commonly assessed expression, maldistribution of income is not an individual characteristic, but is very much a structural aspect of the society or group in which the individual has to function.

The relationship between income and measures of health such as life expectancy is curvilinear. The poorer the group, the sharper and clearer the relationship, but above a certain level of income the curve flattens and the effect of income on health is progressively muted. In terms of country level comparisons, we can note that the effect of income on life expectancy, for example, is stronger in the developing than in the more developed countries.

In a classic series of data produced 25 years ago, Preston developed a family of curves for the relationship between income and life expectancy for different decades of this century. The curves remain qualitatively the same, but over time—as countries prosper—the curves shift, and there is a higher life expectancy for the same income level. This is a most important observation, in that it leads to the view that there are exogenous factors such as technology, both hard and soft, that have contributed to this increase in life expectancy at similar income levels. It is the advent of this technology that has been implicated in the finding of the relatively more rapid improvements in health in many of the developing countries.

As indicated above, it is not only absolute deprivation that is important. As Wilkinson's seminal work has proven, income inequality has an equally and sometimes more powerful influence on such health outcomes as infant mortality rate and life expectancy. Particularly in the developed and richer countries, it is income distribution rather than individual measures of wealth such as per capita GNP that are important. Income maldistribution is associated not only with health outcome but with a whole range of social pathologies. In societies that have more income inequality, there is increased criminal activity, for example.   *interesting*

It has been suggested that it is not only difference in outcomes, such as mortality rates, that can be affected by maldistribution of income. Income differentials result in or are derived from different work opportunities, and these employment differentials are said to create a situation in which the self-worth and autonomy of the lower paid worker are so affected as to lead to varying degrees of psychosocial stress. The spread of information that shows what can be achieved elsewhere makes the appreciation of the gap between aspirations and reality so great that there can be outcomes measured in terms of physiological abnormality. The television images of the rich and famous are seen in the most remote parts of the world, and miracles of modern technology appear to be there simply for the asking. Blood pressure, for example, increases when there is incongruity between what the individual perceives to be an acceptable or conventional lifestyle and that to which he or she is subjected or relegated because of material deprivation.

It also has been proposed that when material deprivation is such that the expectations of the individual cannot be fulfilled, a situation develops similar to the anomie described by Durkheim. As he first conceived it, anomie refers to a state in which the usual norms are no longer clear or observed, and later he used the concept to describe anomic suicide. The competition between individuals and the incongruence between aspirations and possible satisfaction favored the impulse towards suicide. It is not farfetched to relate the increase in criminal activity and social stress attendant upon income inequality to the anomie of Durkheim.

I was intrigued by the possibility that there might be a relationship between income distribution and the rates of suicide. However, in some preliminary analyses of data from our Region, it appears that suicide and death from self-inflicted injury increase as income distribution improves. Countries with more equitable income distribution have higher mortality rates from suicide. This preliminary finding merits more research, as it would seem to run counter to accepted beliefs.

The competitiveness of modern western society stresses and glorifies difference. Wealth may be important not only for its own sake and because it increases options but as a mark of having surpassed others. It satisfies the basic and almost primal drive for recognition. As John Stuart Mill is supposed to have said: ". . . men do not desire to be rich, but to be richer than other men."

I am tempted to assume that there is almost no limit to the degree of income inequality that may occur, and there is evidence that this is worsening, certainly in our hemisphere. Indeed, as Kaus puts it in a provocative book, *The End To Equality*, it may be pointless to seek to reduce income inequality, as there are too many forces pulling in the opposite direction in the liberal, market-based societies that seem

to be overtaking the world. He proposes that it may be more feasible to look for equality in certain civic areas among which he includes health care.

But there are good grounds for believing that there is some theoretical minimum gap in health outcomes for which we can strive in the search for equity. It is possible that health interventions of one or other type may contribute to narrowing this gap. Victora has put forward an interesting thesis based on data collected in Brazil, which show the impact of interventions by the health system in reducing inequities. Any intervention that is likely to improve health will be picked up and used by wealthier groups, with an attendant improvement in their health status. Only after that group has reached what may be considered the maximum plateau will the technology have an effect in improving the health of the poor, thereby closing the gap. There are several factors that contribute to this differential use of the interventions, and they include ease of access to services and the availability and use of information.

It is an interesting phenomenon that the health care interventions that are more equitably used and result in health outcome equity are those that depend on supply and not on demand. The coverage by vaccines is universally high in the Americas, and the success in eliminating diseases such as poliomyelitis has been due to the ability to deliver vaccines to virtually all children. The coverage for polio vaccine in the Americas is about 90% and for BCG, more than 90%. The prospect of eliminating measles by the end of next year is very good because of the possibility of delivering the vaccine to all those who are susceptible. Yet the usage of family planning contraceptives is low—only about two-thirds of the women of childbearing age in Latin America and the Caribbean regularly use contraceptives. The former is essentially supply-driven while the latter is very much dependent on induced demand.

Although we agree that traditional health care services are only partly responsible for health status of the population as a whole, they consume a very large fraction of the nation's health budget and are held to be valuable by all the population. While there is general agreement that in some way there should be equity in terms of health care, there is little agreement as to what that means and how it is to be achieved. Wagstaff is one of the economists who have contributed most perceptively to the debate on equity and health, particularly health care. He points out the need to separate the wish for health care based on altruism from that rooted in a concern for social justice. In exploring the latter, he separates the libertarians, who are concerned with a minimum standard of care for everyone, from the egalitarians, who argue that health care should not be determined by ability to pay, and care should be allocated on the basis of need. It is unlikely that there will ever be consensus, and he argues that there is incompatibility between the three interpretations of equity in health care—"equality of access, allocation according to need and equality of health outcomes." I confess to being philosophically an egalitarian with a preference for allocation of health care according to need as being the best option for ensuring equity of health outcome. Having said that, I am very conscious of the difficulty, if not the impossibility, of finding a definition of a population's needs that is universally acceptable, and I am also aware of the contradiction that sometimes surfaces between the egalitarian posture and the need for efficiency. In addition, even if one adopts a minimalist approach in the sense of a requirement to meet a minimum standard, there is the compounding problem of finding good indicators.

Equity in health care financing is equally complex, and the differentiation is made between vertical equity (whereby payment for care is made according to ability) and horizontal equity (whereby those with the same ability pay the same amounts). I am not sure this distinction is useful in operational or policy terms. The various approaches to financing health care—at least in our Latin American and Caribbean countries—have focused on the need to abolish the segmentation of the funding sources and opt for a more universal system in which the provision of care is separated from the financing. In Latin America there are traditionally three systems of financing health care. There are the ministries of health, the social security institutions, and the private for-profit sector, and there would be general agreement that this arrangement does not lend itself to equitable access to the services that are needed. Perhaps surprisingly, the majority of the expenditure is in the private sector. One of the most thorny issues in our Region is ensuring that health care includes those persons in the informal sector who do not normally pay direct taxes. This informal sector in some countries is larger than the formal one and usually embraces the majority of the poor and especially poor women. Some 25% of the population of Latin America and the Caribbean lack access to basic health services and thus, by definition, there is no universal equity in health care.

We are currently exploring the possibility of micro-insurance schemes for the informal sector, and these will comprise grassroots organizations in areas and populations that are not normally incorporated into the government or private-operated insurance. These schemes, which are usually adapted to the local working or trade situations, are voluntary and preferably run locally, although I believe that their success will depend on at least some initial funding from the state. One of the ways to success of this approach is through having these micro schemes link up in such a manner that there is reasonable sharing of risk.

I have paid more attention to the influence of income or material wealth and health services to equity in health outcomes. This must not be interpreted that I am insensitive to the possibility that differences in other living and working conditions will also impact on health, or that the relative strengths of the various social networks will condition the ability of the individual to retain or recover the healthy state. I am very aware that trying to separate into neat and discrete categories those social factors whose unequal distribution influence health may lead me to fall into the trap of reductionism. We have learnt only too well both in the biological and the social sciences related to health that the systemic approach is the most apt.

If health is universally regarded as a good and there is general agreement on a philosophical level as to the desirability of having equity in terms of health outcomes and equity in terms of access to determinants of health, particularly the health services, why is this so difficult to achieve? First, there would be debate as to whether there can ever be equity in terms of health outcomes and the work of Evans *et al* discusses in detail the basic reasons for there being some differential that can probably never be erased in any society. I have referred to this above. But if the services are organized by human institutions, why is there inequity in terms of availability and access?

Birdsall and her colleagues analyzed this unequal distribution of resources for health in developing countries and described efforts to correct it as "swimming against the tide." She contends that it is based on the distribution of power in these developing societies, although I suspect her analysis is applicable to all societies. If it is governments that are primarily responsible for the allocation or direction of resources, their policies will follow the dictates of rational public choice. This thesis predicates that political decision-makers do not operate simply as individuals seeking to maximize their utility function and to satisfy the perceived needs of individuals. They act to increase the interest, power, and permanence of the group to which they belong, and this approach may be incompatible with equity in access to health services. The recipe for ensuring the reallocation of financing so that the poor benefit equitably from services includes sustained economic growth, political conditions such that there is genuine participation, and gradualism in reallocation to ensure that the resources for the most powerful and articulate groups are

not abruptly reduced. I would lay particular stress on the second condition.

What is the role of organizations such as PAHO and WHO in promoting and making operational the concept of equity in health, especially when our capacity to change the social ecology is limited? I believe that the first and most important task is to promote the collection of the appropriate data and transform them into useful information. It is useless to begin to speak of equity without first having some good measures of the differences that occur. Countries like the United Kingdom, with its long tradition of collection of vital statistics and other health data, are the envy of many of the countries of the developing world. But in addition, we are plagued with the many different systems of data collection that are to be found. A plethora of national institutions may be collecting the same data from individuals without any thought of making them compatible or perhaps organizing fewer systems that are interconnected. It is not uncommon to see the drive of technology producing data in such quantity and of such varying quality that the capacity of the country to analyze them is overwhelmed. Our emphasis is also to stimulate our countries to disaggregate their data so that they may be analyzed in terms of geography, because a country, even the smallest one, is almost a virtual space, and national averages hide the differences that occur. It is critical to have this disaggregation, as it provides information that will permit targeting those areas or groups that are in need, as evidenced by the health data. We are making every effort to stimulate more interest in the traditional vital statistics, which in many places have fallen into neglect, although they were one of, if not the oldest, form of health data to be collected. In addition, it is becoming clearer that any focus on equity demands that the country data sets must go beyond vital statistics and include measures of the performance of the health services as well as other variables such as gender and ethnicity, and a range of social indicators that are usually collected by specific surveys. There has been significant progress, and almost every country of the Americas is now producing basic core data on health as a tool for the planning in the health sector.

Our forte is technical cooperation, which must go beyond assisting in the collection of good data. If we are to help to reduce inequity, we must identify the gaps that occur and target our own technical cooperation towards the application of technologies that may reduce those gaps. In the case of specific diseases, it is conceptually easy to define the gaps or differences between areas or groups and cooperate in the application of the technology that can reduce the gap. As noted above, this is easier with supply-driven interventions, and different tools have to be used in those areas that are essentially demand-driven. Marketing tools and social communication techniques are coming to the fore as behavior change of individuals or groups becomes more and more necessary to impact on the major health problems of our Region. The whole concept of equity of access to the services does not always take account of the fact that accessibility does not necessarily imply usage. The motivation for the socially disadvantaged or excluded to make use of theoretically accessible services may not be the same as for the more fortunate groups, even apart from the difference in transactional costs. The socially disadvantaged are apparently more resistant to changing risk behaviors than others.

I am conscious of the inequity that applies to mental illness. The forms of organization of our mental health services are a manifestation of the frank discrimination against the mentally ill that has its roots and origins in the fear of and ignorance about mental illness. Mental health is rarely included in considerations of public health, perhaps because public health has been linked historically to disease eradication. When I review the many schemes for health sector reform that are currently occupying the attention of our countries, I rarely if ever see any mention of any specific interventions for mental health that ought to be included in the basic or essential package of services that should be made available to all. Perhaps the myth still persists that there are not efficient population-based interventions that can affect the burden of mental illness. In this case the inequity is between groups of persons rather than based on such determinants as place, sex, or race. We believe that this can be changed. We estimate, for example, that the twenty-four million persons in Latin America and the Caribbean with treatable depression who are not receiving regular therapy is evidence of a gap that can be closed. We are convinced that it is perfectly possible to institute treatment schemes at the primary care level that will go some way towards closing this gap.

As those who work for health step forward, I hope that you will make or retain as one of the canons of your faith that it is imperative to advocate as loudly as you can for there to be reduction of those unnecessary and unjust differences that represent inequity. I hope you will see that the widening of the gaps, especially in the areas of social concern, represents a recipe for an unstable world.

BIBLIOGRAPHY

Acheson D. *Independent inquiry into inequalities in health.* Report. London: The Stationary Office; 1998.

Aron R. *Main currents in sociological thought.* Basic Books, Inc; 1967.

Birdsall N, Hecht R. *Swimming against the tide: strategies for improving equity in health.* Washington, D.C. Inter-American Development Bank; 1995. (IDB Working Papers Series No. 305).

Birdsall N, James E. *Efficiency and equity in social spending.* Washington, D.C.: World Bank (Working Papers 1990; Series No. 274).

Black D, et al. *Inequalities in health*: report of a research working group. London: London DHSS; 1980.

Campbell AV. *Medicine, health and justice: the problem of priorities.* Churchill, Livingstone, Edinburgh, London and New York; 1978.

Desjarlais R, Eisenberg L, Good B, Kleinman A. *World mental health*: problems and priorities in low income countries. New York, Oxford: Oxford University Press; 1995.

Dror DM, Jacquier C. *Microinsurance: extending health insurance to the excluded.* International Social Security Review; 1999;52(1):71–97.

Kawachi LS, Miller M, Lasch K, Amich B III. *Income inequality and life expectancy—theory, research and policy.*

Boston: Harvard School of Public Health; 1994. (Society and Health Working Paper Series No. 94-2).

Kohn R, Dohrenwend BP, Mirotiznik J. Epidemiological findings on selected psychiatric disorders in the general population. In: *Adversity, stress and psychopathology*. New York: Oxford University Press; 1998.

Preston SH. *The changing relationship between mortality and level of economic development population*. London; 1975; 231–248.

Renaud M. The future: hygeia versus panakeia? In: *Why some people are healthy and others not? The determinants of health of populations*. Evans RG, Barer ML, Marmor TR. eds. New York: Aldine de Gruyter; 1994.

Rice T. Can markets give us the health system we want? *J Health Politics Policy and Law*. 1997; 22:383–425.

Sigerist HE. *Medicine and human welfare*. New Haven: Yale University Press; 1941.

Victora CG. Reducing health inequalities: can health interventions make an impact? Paper presented at the ninth annual Public Health Forum. London School of Hygiene and Tropical Medicine; April, 1999.

Wagstaff A, Van Doorslaer E. Equity in health care and financing. In: Culyer AJ, Newhouse JP, eds. *North Holland Handbook of Health Economics;* 2000.

Wagstaff A, Van Doorslaer E. Equity in the finance and delivery of health care: concepts and definitions. In: Van Doorslaer E, Wagstaff A, Rutten F, eds. *Equity in finance and delivery of health care: an international perspective*. London: Oxford University Press; 1993.

Whitehead M. *The concepts and principles of equity and health*. Copenhagen: World Health Organization Regional Office for Europe; 1990.

Whitehead M. The health divide. In: Townsend P, Whitehead M, Davidson N, eds. *Inequalities in health: the Black report and the health divide*. 2nd ed. London: Penguin; 1992.

Wilkinson RG. Socio-economic determinants of health: health inequalities: relative or absolute material standards? *Br Med J* 1997; 314:591–595.

Wilkinson RG. *Unhealthy societies: the afflictions of inequality*. London: Routledge; 1996.

Closing the gap is neccessary.

Assessing Equity in Health: Conceptual Criteria

Alexandra Bambas[1] and Juan Antonio Casas[1]

[handwritten: eguality → sameness / equity → fairness]

INTRODUCTION[2]

Fifty years ago, the framers of the Universal Declaration of Human Rights (UDHR) established a benchmark of standards against which to assess equity in health, both in terms of equity in health and well-being and in access to medical care. They wrote:

Article 25. Everyone has the right to a standard of living adequate for the health and well-being of himself and of his family, including food, clothing, housing and medical care and necessary social services, and the right to security in the event of unemployment, sickness, disability, widowhood, old age or other lack of livelihood in circumstances beyond his control.

The UDHR also states:

Article 2. Everyone is entitled to all the rights and freedoms set forth in this Declaration, without distinction of any kind, such as race, colour, sex, language, religion, political or other opinion, national or social origin, property, birth or other status.[3]

Unfortunately, those ideals for human health and well-being set forth in that document have not become a reality for every citizen in the world. In fact, given the competition for resources among different aspects of human well-being, attaining these standards is unfeasible for the present. Consequently, we must now attempt to develop a more organic process for assessing fairness in the distribution of resources for health that takes into consideration our organizational and technical abilities, personal autonomy, and reasonable expectations for action.

In recent decades, important authors have devoted themselves to study, define, and interpret the concepts of equity and social justice, as well as that of health equity. The works of John Rawls,[4] Amartya Sen,[5] and Margaret Whitehead[6] stand out. In our Region, several authors and public health leaders have con-

[1] Division of Health and Human Development, Pan American Health Organization.

[2] This paper is based on a larger work by Alexandra Bambas, entitled "An Interpretation of Equity in Health for Latin America and the Caribbean" (working title), which examines conceptual and programming issues for equity in health in the context of the Region. The paper was also supported by the Division of Health and Human Development's Health Equity Interprogrammatic Group, with inputs from various other PAHO technical units.

[3] The full text of the Universal Declaration of Human Rights is available at: *http://www.ifs.univie.ac.at/intlaw/konterm/vrkon-en/html/doku/humright.htm#1.0.*

[4] Rawls J. A theory of justice. Cambridge: Harvard University Press; 1971.

[5] Sen A. Inequality reexamined. Cambridge: Harvard University Press; 1992.

[6] Whitehead, M (1991) The Concepts and Principles of Equity and Health. World Health Organization, Regional Office for Europe. (Who document EUR/ICP/RPD 414. Unpublished.)

tributed to the understanding of health equity as a public health issue,[7] and since 1995, under the leadership of its Director, Sir George Alleyne, the Pan American Health Organization has identified the reduction of health inequities as the main goal of its technical cooperation.[8] Other leading development institutions, such as the Rockefeller Foundation[9] and the World Bank,[10] also have launched important initiatives that consider health equity as a priority issue for human development.

The persistence of infectious diseases among the poor; the growing proportion of the burden of disease that is due to non-infectious, behavior-related causes; and the growing inequalities within and between countries that have accompanied the globalization process and its worldwide expansion of free trade, market economies, and liberal democracy, have added urgency to the need to address the growing health inequalities. As a result, national and international health authorities have increasingly addressed the macrodeterminants of health inequities. The issue of health inequities and their relation to living conditions is now in the mainstream of public health thinking. And yet, although the technical aspects of measuring inequalities in health have evolved, insufficient attention is given to the explanation of why inequalities in health or health resources might be unfair or what the larger implications of labeling them as unfair might be. Moreover, the term "equity" often is used loosely, making it unclear as to how the term should be interpreted in a given context.

Many of the discussions about health equity make reasonable claims that there are inequalities in health status and access to care for different categories of people, whether identified by social class (as measured by income, wealth, and/or formal education), spatial distribution, gender, or ethnicity. Those who work in the public policy sector take this a step further, often referring to these inequalities in health as inequities, casually using the term as shorthand for describing differences between better- and worse-off groups. Implicit to these discussions is an assumption that any difference is unacceptable and requires attention and intervention, but such discussions rarely provide an explanation for that value judgment or make distinctions between different kinds and levels of inequalities.

Asserting that these inequalities are inequities makes a forceful claim about justice—the normative implication of the word is useful. Confusing "equity" with "equality," a common implication of comparisons between the best-off and worst-off, can result in a much higher standard than we might agree to under a more careful examination, however. The failure to distinguish between philosophical and pragmatic decisions regarding equity concerns in health could confuse the assessment of resource allocation or other policy decisions. This, in turn, would undermine the transparency of the process, making it difficult to generate public support.

At least three emerging empirical findings commonly drive the claim that inequalities in health between socioeconomic groups should be a development issue, and specifically a public health concern, particularly in Latin America and the Caribbean.

1. The poor use fewer public resources than middle and upper income groups.
2. There are vast and patterned health inequalities between socioeconomic groups, as well as between gender and ethnic origin categories, suggesting links between

[7] These Latin American public health figures include, but are not limited to, Jaime Breilh, Juan Cesar Garcia, Asa Cristina Laurell, Cristina Possas, Mario Testa, Naomar de Almeida Filho, Pedro Luis Castellanos, Juan Samaja, Carlos Montoya, Jeanette Vega, among others.

[8] See for example, Pan American Health Organization. *Annual report of the Director, 1995: In search of equity.* Official document No. 277. Washington, DC: 1996; and Alleyne G.A.O. "Equity and Health," speech presented at the XI World Congress of Psychiatry, Hamburg, Germany, August 1999.

[9] Rockefeller Foundation. Global health equity initiative report. In press.

[10] The current work by Davidson Gwatkin and Adam Wagstaff in the Poverty and Health Interprogrammatic Group in the World Bank is of particular importance.

health outcomes and a variety of material and social living conditions.

3. Inequalities in the impact of these macro-determinants on health and overall well-being are growing.

These observations are often associated with the effects of globalization, and imply that intervention is required to prevent market distributions of resources from creating large discrepancies in health. These concerns also suggest that past interventions have not sufficiently compensated for these market effects.

DEFINITIONS OF EQUITY

Dictionary definitions of "equity" are fairly consistent. The term is defined as "justice according to natural law or right; specifically, freedom from bias or favoritism," or "the state, ideal, or quality of being just, impartial, and fair."[11]

"Inequity," then, is the linguistic opposite: the state, ideal, or quality of being unjust, partial, or unfair. Most importantly, notice that not *equality of distributions* but rather *fairness of distributions* is central to the definition. Although "equality" and "equity" are often conflated, the words have two distinct meanings and are conceptually very different. Equality is sameness, and equity is fairness. In any particular situation, equal may not be equitable, or equal may be precisely equitable, but we must present an ethical justification for why a certain distribution constitutes an inequity.

Vertical and Horizontal Equity

In describing an equitable situation, distinctions must be made between the appropriateness of equal and unequal distributions—or horizontal and vertical equity—either of which may constitute "even-handed treat-

ment," depending on the situation. Equity simultaneously requires that relevantly similar cases be treated in similar ways, and relevantly different cases be treated in different ways. As noted in the *Dictionary of Philosophy*, controversy arises from the delineation of relevant similarity—*horizontal equity* is the allocation of equal or equivalent resources for *equal need; vertical equity* is the allocation of different resources for *different levels of need.*

These two conceptions of equity have dramatically different policy implications and cannot be applied randomly to problems. Rather, their application must appeal to some principle or special feature of the problem that justifies the choice of one over the other. For example, a universal health care plan might appeal to horizontal equity on the basis that *everyone* needs health care at some point. On the other hand, targeted programs for the poor would appeal to vertical equity. The distinction between these situations turns on the interpretation of *need*: in the first case, the justification is that everyone needs health care in the biological sense, while the second case appeals to a sense of financial need of the poor which doesn't apply to the non-poor.

Vertical equity has a higher potential for redistributing resources, and therefore often faces more political obstacles. However, in the current political climate, which challenges the legitimacy of public provision of services in areas thought to have market potential, vertical equity has gained momentum as a mechanism for constraining claims of need to those based on severe financial deprivation. For instance, where market mechanisms have been introduced into national health systems in the process of health sector reform, publicly funded basic packages or focalization strategies were instituted to provide for the needs of the worst-off. This approach has been criticized as having an overly narrow interpretation of need, which left large segments of the population vulnerable once again. On the other hand, some focalized strategies based on vertical equity are seen as quite reasonable and successful, such as in immunization programs.

---

[11] Webster's New Collegiate Dictionary; American Heritage Dictionary.

EQUITY IN ACCESS TO
HEALTH CARE SERVICES

An operational definition of health equity that focuses on need as the appropriate distribution mechanism specifically addresses equity in access to health care services. Aday's definition,[12] which has pervaded thinking in the health field, often is taken for granted and seldom questioned. Aday et al. define an "equitable distribution of health-care services" as "one in which illness (as defined by the patient and his family or by health-care professionals) is the major determinant of the allocation of resources."

The crux of the argument is that health resources are special goods that should not be distributed strictly as normal market commodities according to economic resources, because their social worth is significant. But this service-oriented approach has been found to be insufficient in reducing inequalities in health status and access to health between socioeconomic groups, a finding cited by the widely influential Black and Acheson Reports of the United Kingdom. These reports examined the British National Health System, a prime example of universal coverage in health, and concluded that the effect of approaching health using a medical services strategy did not address concerns of reducing health inequalities and achieving fairness.

"Access to medical services" historically has been used as a measure of fair distribution, partly because it is easier to measure and to improve access to services than to achieve more ambitious goals—say, securing a certain level of well-being in a population—and because of the historical compartmentalization of the social sectors within government, which provide focal advantages, but may at times limit the activities seen as appropriate for any one sector.

Additionally, there is an implicit assumption that services are a means to improve the

population's health, an assumption that has not been sufficiently confirmed.[13] Recent attention to inequalities in health status, especially with regard to socioeconomic categories, underlies a certain dissatisfaction with approaches strictly focused on access to services. This is due in part to the recognition that medical services may not be the most important determinant of health status and certainly are not the only means to improving health status. Insofar as access to services is supposed to be a means to higher level goals, such as better health, or even more opportunities in life, it is a limited measure of health equity. Various other sectors and aspects of life affect one's health status, including living conditions, working conditions, environmental issues such as air quality, education level, and access to cultural, social, and political participation.

By limiting our evaluation of health equity to "access to medical services," we ignore the importance of other sectors in determining health, and effectively exclude their incorporation into an equity strategy. Such an approach tends to value these services for their own sake, rather than emphasizing the role of medical services as *one of many means* to attain health.

If our consideration of health equity is widened to include inequalities in health outcomes, it becomes necessary to measure health status directly (rather than using only access to services) and to incorporate the analysis of access to other basic services and the level of satisfaction of other basic needs into the assessment of equity in health. The shift from a medical services approach to a health outcomes approach involves the recognition that people do not get sick randomly, but in relation to their living, working, environmental, social, and political contexts, as well as with regard to biological and environmental factors that are unevenly distributed in the popula-

[12] Aday LA and Andersen RM (1981). Equity of access to medical care: a conceptual and empirical review. *Med Care* 1981; 19 (12), Suppl. pp. 4–27.

[13] McKeon T. The role of medicine: dream, miracle or nemesis? Nuffield Provincial Trust; 1976 (also available in Spanish, under the title, "El papel de la medicina: sueño, espejismo o nemesis." México: Siglo XXI; 1982).

are available 4-7

tion. This broader concept is also much more conducive to considering the improvement of health status as part of the larger work of human development.

EQUITY IN HEALTH OUTCOMES

Based on the broad concept of health equity, as developed by Margaret Whitehead and adopted by EURO/WHO, the government of the United Kingdom has taken the policy position that all health differences between the best-off and worst-off in different socioeconomic groups constitute inequities in health. Whitehead defines health inequities as "differences in health which are not only unnecessary and avoidable but, in addition, are considered unfair and unjust."[14]

If this were the complete definition, people with different life perspectives and even different political ideologies might be able to agree to it in principle, which would make it useful in the larger political forum to generate a working consensus on the matter. However, it entails reaching agreement on two potentially controversial parameters, i.e., determining what is unnecessary and unfair vis-à-vis what is inevitable and unavoidable.

Whitehead goes on to specify seven determinants of health inequalities that can be identified:

not considered unfair or unjust

1. Natural, biological variation. *unfair or unjust*
2. Health damaging behavior that is freely chosen, such as participation in certain sports and pastimes.
3. The transient health advantage of one group over another when that group is first to adopt a health-promoting behavior (as long as other groups have the means to catch up fairly soon).

4. Health damaging behavior in which the degree of choice of lifestyles is severely restricted.
5. Exposure to unhealthy, stressful living and working conditions.
6. Inadequate access to essential health and other basic services.
7. Natural selection or health-related social mobility involving the tendency for sick people to move down the social scale.

Health inequalities determined by the first three categories would not be considered unfair nor unjust, while the last four would be considered by many to be avoidable and the resultant health differences to be unjust."[15]

Although Whitehead's definition includes adequate access to health services as a condition of justice, it extends far beyond that—and beyond the more procedural standard related to access to services—to a much broader set of conditions that can affect health and establish a health advantage of one group over another. It's a robust concept of equity, encompassing a range of situations including outcomes, exposures, risks, living conditions, and social mobility.

CRITERIA FOR ASSESSING HEALTH EQUITY

The burden of proof lies in demonstrating that a situation is inequitable (rather than equitable), because making a social argument to change the present order requires justifying the allocation of public resources for interventions to redress the inequality. But to make this claim, we must give contextual and concrete meaning to the operational definitions of equity to determine when the judgment would apply. These meanings are reflected in the criteria that are repeatedly referred to in discussions regarding fair distributions of goods.

---

[14] Whitehead M (1991) The Concepts and Principles of Equity and Health. World Health Organization, Regional Office for Europe (WHO document EUR/ICP/RPD 414. Unpublished); p. 5.

[15] Whitehead M (1991) The Concepts and Principles of Equity and Health. World Health Organization, Regional Office for Europe (WHO document EUR/ICP/RPD 414. Unpublished); p. 6.

exosmog in city [handwritten margin note]

To establish a situation as inequitable, differences in distributions of a good, such as health resources or even the larger determinants of health status, must satisfy each of the criteria:

determinants of inequity [handwritten margin note]

- The differences in distribution must be *avoidable*,
- must *not reflect free choice*, and
- the claim must link the distribution to a *responsible agent*.

As the claimants, we must be able to argue how these criteria relate to particular claims of inequity.

Although these criteria might be applied to either individual distributions or to social distributions, their implications will take on somewhat different tones with each. For the purposes of policy development, we are concerned with social distributions, and therefore the interpretation of each of these criteria will relate not to equity judgments of any particular person's situation, but to trends in the health of the population and its subgroups. Some might argue that distributions are *politically necessary*—that sufficient support cannot be generated to support redistribution. But political will should be driven by justice; it should not constrain justice. If political will is lacking but equity criteria are present, mobilizing civil society to create political pressure becomes a technical issue.

Avoidability

"Avoidability" is a key criterion for equity, because if a distribution is not avoidable, it cannot be interpreted to be unfair in a social sense. While we emotionally respond by feeling that the universe or life is not just—and we may even have a will to intervene to change such distributions—to make a social claim based on equity is quite a different matter in that it *requires* action.

A proposal for redistribution, whether it be of health services or of macro-determinants of health, must show the current distribution to be avoidable in several senses.

It must be *technically avoidable* because current scientific and organizational knowledge provides a solution for successful intervention.

It must be *financially avoidable* because sufficient resources exist either within the public sector or more generally to satisfy fair conditions.

And it must be *morally avoidable* because the proposed redistribution would not violate some other, greater, sense of justice.

The subcategories of avoidability are highly relevant to claims of socioeconomic health inequities. Certainly there are individual cases of "technically unavoidable" health differences, such as in the case of health harms linked to naturally occurring genetic variations. But unless given reason to believe the contrary, we would not expect such occurrences to be patterned according to socioeconomic groups, thereby eliminating one source of "technically unavoidable" health inequalities and strengthening claims that patterned distributions of health may constitute inequities. Assuming that genetically related differences in health are not used to define our groups, the health standard of best-off groups demonstrates that those health indicators are indeed technically feasible. That is, in *technical terms* there is no reason why all groups could not achieve health levels similar to those of best-off groups.

However, the setting of standards according to best-off groups may be prohibitively expensive, at least above a certain level of health. Diminishing margins of utility certainly do not argue against *any* redistribution or investment, but may place a limit on what might be financially possible in reducing health inequalities given resource constraints. Therefore, such studies contribute significantly to our understanding of financial avoidability, and therefore to reasonable and fair differences, even if absolute equality proves unfeasible. Finally, the evaluation of financial feasibility and the effect of re-distributions cannot be restricted to current public spending levels, but must necessarily include an economic evaluation of the availability of external resources based on the potential to increase fiscal base, since the question at issue is whether the financial resources exist at a macroeconomic level, not only within the institutional confines of the health sector.

At some point, we may determine that a certain redistribution level is technically and financially feasible, but impinges on other social values to the extent that the redistribution itself becomes unjust, either by severely restricting civil liberties or by prioritizing health to the unjustifiable detriment of other social goods. Analyses must therefore include not only studies of diminishing margins of utility, but also the larger social effect of such redistributions. Hypothetically, if, for a given country, we found that we could bring inequalities of infant mortality rates, maternal mortality rates, and communicable diseases within "an acceptable range" only by instituting tax rates of 90% of income, we may decide that personal freedoms would be compromised to an extent that the social injustices created are greater than those that existed under conditions of larger health inequalities. If we accomplished the task by directing public spending for health activities by virtually eliminating other important national programs, not only might we find greater injustices than health inequalities, but also the actions might prove counter-productive if certain other programs (such as education or environmental protection) were to be affected.

If an argument that inequities exist is able to respond to each of these issues, it has succeeded in establishing that such inequalities are in fact avoidable, perhaps the most difficult of the criteria to secure.

Choice

Choice is particularly relevant to interpreting justice in health in terms of the protection of individual autonomy. Therefore, *health behaviors* are better at indicating possible choice issues than are health outcomes. The application of choice as a criterion might range from an individual electing to (1) engage in an activity, to (2) buy a product, and to (3) prioritize needs. We hope that given sufficient information and opportunity, people will opt for activities and behaviors that enhance their health. Even when such activities and behaviors may not always be chosen, justifying health-enhancing interventions may be limited by concerns for autonomy and the preservation of civil liberties.

Free choices may, in fact, create acceptable differences between *individuals'* health, as some persons may choose behavior that leads to worse health outcomes. But if the choice was in fact made under perfect, or even reasonably high conditions of choice, including adequate information and free will, claims of an injustice would be more difficult to sustain.

Particularly in the context of population-based analyses, however, protecting autonomy and promoting health often are more complimentary goals rather than competing interests. While individuals might make free choices based on their own particular wants or needs, we would not expect to see strong patterns of such behavior stratified in socioeconomic groups, unless an additional correlation that explains the concentration of risky behavior were presented.

A case for socioeconomic inequities in health must be built on the presumption that population *groups* would not freely choose lesser levels of health. In fact, some studies have shown that health behaviors do not differ significantly between population groups, and when they do, such as in the case of high fat diets among some minority groups in the United States or the urban poor in Latin America and the Caribbean, culture and lack of health information can be seen to clearly diminish the role of free choice. Further, when health behaviors are controlled for income, differences between groups dissolve, and income is not usually considered a "chosen" socioeconomic category. Consequently, choice as a justification for health differences tends to fall away in population studies. Therefore, when we do see such patterns, there is reason to believe that low levels of choice, or a thin sense of choice, might better describe those behaviors or decisions. Investigation into causality, whether through physical or social science, can bolster the argument that choice is limited.

Opponents of redistribution sometimes try to limit the scope of challenges to choice by depending on claims of economic choices in prioritizing goods or procedural interpretations of legal entitlement (in the case of public programs) as sufficient conditions for establishing free choice. Such conclusions generally rely on assumptions of equal opportunity for individuals within a society, at least at some level, although little attention is given to elaborating on the conditions of equal opportunity or a practical demonstration that such opportunity exists. Failure of the poor to "protect their health," for instance, is seen as due to their own negligence or to the life situation that they have put themselves in (e.g. "choosing" to work in a dangerous factory), rather than any larger social, economic, or political disadvantages over which they had little control.

Some might argue that the poor or other vulnerable groups "choose" poor health, particularly when they fail to seek care when they are ill. However, the priorities that intervene to prevent such utilization of care are often not only equally basic and necessary for survival, but also often contribute to the family's health in some other way, as when financial resources are used to purchase food or support the survival of the family business. Such arguments gain by conflating "decision making," which can include prioritizing certain needs over other needs, with a richer meaning of "free choice." Further, if we can demonstrate that health is strongly linked to other social sectors, the argument that the poor can "choose" to invest in health by financially prioritizing health care services over, say, housing or nutrition, loses its weight, since the areas are interrelated, and that "choice" simply becomes a decision, with little real meaning in terms of improving one's well-being.

Insofar as access to health services is concerned, proponents of resource redistribution have succeeded in expanding the narrow, but commonly used interpretation of "choice"— the *legal right to utilize resources*. They include more socially embedded issues that are needed to access health resources, such as support services, including transportation. Recognizing the social context of a situation demonstrates how real "choices" can be thwarted by the reality of people's daily lives. Removal of those barriers, then, actually enhances individual autonomy in a meaningful sense, rather than detracting from it.

Transportation is only one of many barriers to free choice. While individuals often do make choices about their own health, decisions also are made by groups at the national, community, and family levels. Such situations can be used against the politically disenfranchised in a democracy, if the assertion is made that all citizens have agreed to certain conditions, and therefore have "chosen" those conditions. The recognition of macrodeterminants of health, including social and economic factors that influence health status, has greatly broadened the social meaning of health resources, and consequently has expanded the list of relevant resources involved in the choice claim. Lack of access to education and access to information, for instance, can ground a health inequity claim related to choice. Though more difficult to empirically demonstrate, psychological issues also are basic to a conception of choice. Elements of social control and influence, actual and perceived locus of control, and the larger implications of certain health-related choices on one's life become very important to identify in order to establish that choice is more limited than it might appear.

Agency

The third criterion for establishing that an inequity exists is that the claim be linked to a *responsible agent*. To make this determination, either of two meanings of "responsible" may be used. We may establish that there is a *culpable* entity who caused direct or indirect harm, as we might apply in cases of damage to health due to environmental degradation or occupational hazards. One of the difficulties in identifying and establishing the culpable agent is that culpability can be masked. The externalization of health harms in industry or manufacturing, for instance, would first have to be recognized, then traced. In the absence of empirical studies linking problems to their sources, our ability to perceive the culpability of a particular agent will be impaired, even if there is a very direct cause/effect relationship. Further, for the purposes of socioeconomic differences in health, discrete instances of culpability are less relevant than larger systematic patterns of harms that would be generated through responses to policy, or its absence.

Alternatively, we might make a claim that there is an *accountable* entity, one who is responsible for rectifying the unfair distribution. In the case of health equity, claims often center on the responsibility of the government to ensure certain rights or provide a certain amount of protection to all citizens, which justifies state intervention. A claim of lax or unenforced government regulations, or governmental assistance in externalizing health harms, makes a particularly strong claim. Although a government might not be responsible for creating a health-harming situation, once an issue has been publicly discussed, lack of response by government must be interpreted as a decision affecting the public to which it, as a presumably just institution, must be held accountable. The level of governance then, will also affect perceptions of the responsibility (and the ability to respond) of the government.

The Spectrum of Inequalities

If any one of these criteria is absent, or is present only weakly, the argument that a difference is an inequity begins to lose power. In addition to the empirical verification that inequalities in health status or access to resources exist, scientific research can assist in

demonstrating that these criteria apply, thereby greatly strengthening the political claim that inequities also exist. Because scientific knowledge is constantly growing, our interpretation of whether criteria apply to specific issues also changes over time. For instance, in relation to "free choice," alcoholism and smoking are not seen as much as lifestyle *choices* as they once were, because of increasing evidence on the biological basis of addiction. Social science research also contributes to our interpretations, as when we attend to the effect of targeted advertising on alcohol consumption and smoking rates.

When we make the claim that differences in health are inequitable, the strength of the evidence or the argument, according to the above criteria, will determine the level of inequity. We might think of this as a spectrum, with each of the criteria moving our assessment of the situation either closer to "misfortune" or to "inequity."

Misfortune	Inequities
(Fair differences)	(Unfair differences)
Avoidable Differences	
Chosen Differences	
Responsible Agent	

To be sure, we must be willing to recognize some differences as "fair" differences; otherwise, the criteria would not be meaningful. Genetic birth defects and deaths due to "old age" may be very unfortunate but not necessarily unfair if little could have been done to prevent them; that is, they were not avoidable. Therefore, it will also be important for a clear analysis to identify those differences that do not fit into the criteria.

CONCLUSION

The framework presented here must now be supplemented with quantitative and qualitative information that applies each of these criteria to the health conditions and broader societal abilities and resources in order to set priorities and targets for equity in health. Research must be supported not only by traditional epidemiological studies but also by social health research, including methodologies that are continuing to be developed. The particular resources and challenges will differ among countries, and the quest for health equity should be recognized as a development process, and one that must alter its goals on occasion to adjust to the changing environment.

An equity-driven approach in health policy requires a broad vision of the determinants of population health and an understanding of how both health policy and wider social policy will affect those determinants. To the extent that health and other socioeconomic factors are interdependent, health policy must consider how other sectoral policies and actions, as well as societal trends, can be directed to promote health equity. Similarly, health policy must take into consideration how health policy can contribute to broader equity goals in health development.

Finally, the pursuit of equity is necessarily linked to issues of governance, which include accountability, transparency, decision-making procedures, and the ability of the political arena to allow for broad representation and the effective exercise of choice by all social groups and members of society.[16] Leadership in health equity requires both a high capability for managing resources and developing policy and a strong political society. Once a society embraces a political foundation of egalitarianism, whereby all citizens of a country are due equal regard under the law and have equal political voices, societies themselves become the ultimate arbitrators of equity, in health or any other sphere.

we need this

[16] Gilson L. In defence and pursuit of equity. *Soc Sci Med* 1998; 47: 1891–1896.

Could be prevented = avoidable

HEALTH DISPARITIES IN LATIN AMERICA AND THE CARIBBEAN: THE ROLE OF SOCIAL AND ECONOMIC DETERMINANTS

Juan Antonio Casas,[1] J. Norberto W. Dachs,[1] and Alexandra Bambas[1]

The Latin American and Caribbean (LAC) region demonstrates the greatest disparities in income and in other socioeconomic determinants of health. Although research in many developed countries has provided strong evidence on the extent and strength of the relationships between these determinants and health, relatively little has been established on this relationship in the context of the countries in LAC. Nevertheless, available evidence shows that the distributions of health status and access to health services among different socioeconomic groups follow patterns that place the most vulnerable groups in situations of continuing and often growing disadvantage.

Evidence also shows that such social and economic advantages are more strongly related to health outcomes than are need-based allocations of health services. This is a particular problem in LAC, where disparities in socioeconomic factors have continued to increase since 1980. Although general health has improved in LAC countries, gains in health status have not been made equally among various socioeconomic groups. Overall health improvement does not imply diminishing disparities either between or within countries. Rather, improvements appear to be disproportionately weighted toward those who already have a greater share of social and economic advantages in society, while the health of disadvantaged groups improves less consistently and at much more modest rates.

HEALTH AND THE SOCIAL AND ECONOMIC CONTEXT OF LATIN AMERICA AND THE CARIBBEAN

National health statistics in LAC have shown improvement over the past 35 to 50 years for almost all health indicators, including life expectancy, infant mortality, the incidence of many communicable diseases, and vaccination coverage, to name a few. For example:

- Life expectancy over the last 35 years has followed the worldwide trend for the 20th century, rising from 56.9 to 68.5 years, an increase of almost 12 years.[2] During this time, specific mortality rates for almost all age groups and in all countries showed significant reductions.[3]

[1] Division of Health and Human Development, Pan American Health Organization. The authors wish to acknowledge other members of PAHO's Division of Health and Human Development who made significant comments to this paper, including Elsa Gómez, Edward Greene, Cristina Torres, and Raúl Molina.

[2] There are exceptions in a few countries, specifically in the groups between 20 and 39 years of age for males, due to AIDS and violent deaths.

[3] Murray CJL, Chen LC. In search of a contemporary theory for understanding mortality change. *Soc Sci Med* 1993; 35 (2): 143–145.

- Although life expectancy in LAC in 1990–1994 (68.5) was still below that of North America (76.2) and Western Europe (80.2), it was above the world average of 64.3 years and above that of Africa (51.8) and Asia (64.5), but below that for eastern Asia (69.7).
- Similarly, the infant mortality rate in LAC has dropped from 125 per 1,000 live births in 1950–1955 to 36 in 1995–2000.[4]

The range of national health levels among countries around the world broadened for most health statistics, however, revealing a growing gap between the extremes of the global social ladder. Improvements in life expectancy in the LAC region are not keeping pace with those of other regions. If we compare LAC countries to East Asian countries, their relative life expectancies at the beginning of the 1960s were 56.9 and 51.4, respectively; currently these values are 68.5 and 69.7. In other words, whereas LAC enjoyed a five-year advantage in life expectancy over East Asia thirty years ago it now lags by 1.2 years.[5]

Improvements in health also have been uneven within LAC and do not correspond to the region's economic development level. Successes in the reduction of infant mortality by countries such as Costa Rica, Cuba, and Chile, which have diverse political and economic circumstances, demonstrate that most LAC countries have not yet tapped their potential to improve population health.[6]

The level of population health, particularly over long periods of time, tends to be associated with a level of economic growth and overall availability of resources, as is evident when a health indicator such as the infant mortality rate is correlated with per capita income (see Figure 1). Countries and social groups that have higher incomes usually have better health conditions and better overall living con-

FIGURE 1. Correlation between the infant mortality rate and the per capita income (PPP), selected countries in the Americas, 1996.

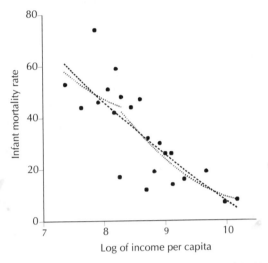

Source: Pan American Health Organization/Division of Health and Human Development and United Nations Development Program/*Human Development Report, 1997*

ditions since they have more economic and technological resources to fulfill basic needs. The political context also is an important determinant of health. With few exceptions, those countries in the world that developed institutions of democratic governance and strong civil societies usually have established long-term social policies that tend towards a broader distribution of income and social benefits. Interestingly, the countries that applied social policies providing their populations with better access to education, basic health services, nutrition, and basic sanitation have achieved low mortality rates compared to countries of equal or even better economic performance, but where large disparities of income and resources persist.[7]

These epidemiological transitions have occurred within a context of rapidly changing economic and social conditions. In LAC during the 1990s, the macroeconomic adjustment policies adopted at the beginning of the decade generally have led to economic growth

---

[4] United Nations. *World population prospects, 1998 revision*. New York, NY: UN; 1998.

[5] United Nations. *World population prospects, 1996 revision*. New York, NY: UN; 1996.

[6] Pan American Health Organization. *Health statistics from the Americas, 1992 edition*. Washington, DC: PAHO; 1992.

[7] Wilkinson RG. *Unhealthy societies: the afflictions of inequality*. London: Routledge; 1996.

recovery, increased exports, substantially higher levels of direct foreign investment, and an increase in total public expenditure since the crisis of the early 1980s.

Although social sector spending has now exceeded the pre-crisis spending levels as a percent of GDP, the Economic Commission for Latin America and the Caribbean (ECLAC) points out some sobering facts: spending levels vary significantly between countries, with some countries spending at levels significantly below pre-crisis levels; a "very large" percentage of the increase in social funding is spent on social security (specifically on pension benefits, which is the least progressive item in distributional terms); and spending on human capital, such as education and health care, has increased less than figures would indicate.[8]

Overall economic growth also has not led to decreases in income disparities between families:

• The Region of the Americas has been identified as having the most unequal distribution of income in the world; the Gini coefficient for Latin America is estimated at 0.49, compared to 0.44 for Africa, 0.32 for East Asia, and 0.31 for Southeast Asia, with Brazil, Guatemala, and Honduras leading the way as the most skewed in terms of income concentration among the better off.
• In some countries in LAC the wealthiest 10% of the population receives 84 times the income received by the poorest 10%.[9]
• A World Bank study of 102 developing countries in the world found that the poverty levels in 15 of the 17 LAC countries studied were four times that of other countries with similar income levels.[10]

Further, the poor are falling further behind regarding income distribution, as the wealthiest sector of the population captures most of the benefits of economic growth:

• Between 1980 and 1989, the Gini coefficient rose for almost every country in Latin America, with Costa Rica as the only generally agreed-upon exception to growing income inequalities.[11]
• In 1995, the purchasing power parity of the richest 1% (with $66,363 per capita per year) and the poorest 1% (with $159 per capita per year) of the Latin American population reached 417, higher than at any time in recorded history, and likely has worsened since then.[12]
• In Brazil, which has the highest income disparity in the world, the proportion of the total national income of the poorest half of the population decreased between 1960 and 1990 from 18% to 12%, while the income of the richest 20% of the population increased from 54% to 65% of total national income.[13]

While the proportion of income captured by the wealthy grows, a large proportion of the population continues to be trapped in poverty:

• Poverty rates in LAC are not improving: the poverty rate in 1980 was 35%, topping 40% for the 1990–1994 period, before falling to 35% in 1997.
• With the population's demographic growth, the number of people living in poverty in LAC has increased over the last two decades, reaching roughly 200 million within Latin America in 1997.[14]

[8] Ocampo JA. Income distribution, poverty and social expenditure in Latin America. Paper prepared for the first Conference of the Americas convened by the Organization of American States. Washington, DC: 6 March 1998. Found at http://www.eclac.cl/english/Coverpage/oeaningles.htm.
[9] Interamerican Development Bank. Economic and social progress in Latin America, 1998–1999 report: Facing up to inequality in Latin America. Washington, DC: IADB; 1999.
[10] World Bank in Kliksberg B. Inequality in Latin America: A key issue. Washington, DC: INDES IADB; 1998.

[11] Kliksberg B. Inequality in Latin America: A key issue. Washington, DC: INDES IADB; 1998.
[12] Londoño and Szkeley, in Kliksberg B. Inequality in Latin America: A key issue. Washington, DC: INDES IADB; 1998.
[13] Kliksberg B. Inequality in Latin America: A key issue. Washington, DC: INDES IADB; 1998.
[14] Economic Commission for Latin America and the Caribbean. Panorama social de America Latina. Santiago, Chile: ECLAC; 1998.

Gini coefficient
0 = perfect equality
1 = totally inequality

- The rate of extreme poverty was the same in 1997 as in 1980, around 15%, which translates to more than 100 million people.[15]
- If income distribution in LAC had not worsened since 1980, the increase in poverty between 1983 and 1995 would have been half of what it was.[16]

Although current poverty rates are comparable to those of twenty years ago, the geographic distribution of poverty has changed considerably:

- Rapid urbanization of the population has increased the proportion of urban dwellers who are poor from 25% in 1980 to 34% in 1994; the urban poor now comprise the larger portion of the desperately poor in the Region.
- More than half of the population in extreme poverty now lives in cities, whereas only one-third of the people living in extreme poverty lived in urban areas in 1990.
- The percentage of the rural population living in poverty has changed very little, hovering between 53% and 56% from 1980 to 1994.[17]
- Some countries have suffered even more severe poverty increases. For instance, the poverty rate in Trinidad and Tobago increased from 3.5% of the households in 1980 to almost 15% in 1990, and it is estimated that the poverty rate has exceeded 20% in the mid-1990s.

The urbanization of poverty in LAC is strongly linked to persistent structural unemployment and the marginal nature of most new economic activities:

- Even in a country such as Chile, with a relatively modern economic structure, more than half of new employment in the decade has taken place in the informal sector of the economy, which has a negative impact on social protection, stability, and long-term development.[18]
- The ILO estimated that, during the 1990s, eight of every ten new jobs in LAC have been in poor-quality occupations within the informal sector.[19]

SOURCES OF DATA/LITERATURE FOR THE ANALYSIS OF DETERMINANTS OF DISPARITIES IN HEALTH IN THE REGION

Research conducted in the United States, Canada, and Western Europe over the past two decades has given increasing importance to the study and understanding of the relations between living conditions and health, focusing on disparities. A bibliographic database on this topic, prepared by PAHO's Division of Health and Human Development,[20] includes more than four thousand entries, with most of the empirical information based on situations in developed countries. The concern with this area has now reached what could be called the mainstream public health literature in the United States and Europe, and public health oriented institutions are calling to broaden the parameters of the health policy debate to include economic and social issues.

The body of knowledge dealing with levels of socioeconomic disparities and their effect on health is significantly smaller for those areas of the world whose socioeconomic conditions are lower than those in the developed

[15] Inter-American Development Bank. *Economic and social progress in Latin America, 1998–1999 report: Facing up to inequality in Latin America.* Washington, DC: IADB; 1999.

[16] Birdsall N, Londoño L. Asset inequality matters: An assessment of the World Bank's approach to poverty reduction. *American Economist Review* 1997; 5.

[17] Economic Commission for Latin America and the Caribbean. *Panorama social de America Latina.* Santiago, Chile: ECLAC; 1998.

[18] World Bank. *Labor and economic reforms in Latin America and the Caribbean.* Washington, DC: World Bank; 1995.

[19] International Labour Organization. Labour overview, 1997. Lima, Regional Office for Latin America and the Caribbean; 1997.

[20] Wing SB, Richardson D. Material living conditions and health in the United States, Canada and Western Europe: Review of recent literature and bibliography. Washington, DC: Pan American Health Organization; 1999. (Research in public health technical papers #9).

countries, particularly LAC. PAHO also has completed a similar bibliographical review to document the body of literature on socioeconomic disparities in health that has been produced within LAC, and found only 304 documents, many of which are unpublished.[21]

In addition to the paucity of information, the literature was found to have other limitations, such as:

- Much of the literature addresses philosophical and theoretical considerations rather than empirical information that can provide evidence for action;
- Studies address narrow age groups, and there is an absence of studies relating to adult health in particular;
- Results are often unreliable due to flaws in data quality, design, or analysis; and
- Very few studies have been conducted at the local level with primary data collection.

Despite the limited number of studies focusing specifically on the Region, it is clear that the disparities in health outcomes and access to care between various socioeconomic groups and geographic populations in LAC have remained large in the past few decades, even tending to increase in many cases. Disparities in health status and access/utilization of health services between better- and worse-off groups according to socioeconomic criteria manifest themselves by almost any criterion of classification used.

There is most evidence for the socioeconomic category of income, and several studies have documented the differences between the poor and non-poor in health outcomes and access to health services.

Although these studies' findings may appear intuitive, documenting these findings through empirical observation not only strengthens the case for socioeconomic dis-

parities in health, but also provides more complete information for the analysis of these health issues. One of the difficulties of interpreting these studies is that individuals in vulnerable populations are often vulnerable on several counts. The categorical associations presented below are not controlled for other socioeconomic factors; they are simply correlations, without explicit evidence for causality.

The socioeconomic categories, as well as the health indicators, were chosen as study topics primarily because sufficient empirical information exists for the described population to establish the correlation. In addition to primary data collection, many studies use data from Living Standards Measurement Surveys (LSMS) and Demographic Health Surveys (DHS), which have proven to be valuable, if incomplete, information sources. An example of this approach is the recently completed IHEP-EquiLAC Initiative, carried out by PAHO (Division of Health and Human Development) in collaboration with UNDP, IADB and the World Bank, some of the findings of which are mentioned below,[22] along with other results from both published and unpublished literature.

HEALTH INEQUALITIES AMONG COUNTRIES

Although health indicators have generally improved in every country, significant disparities persist between countries. Further, improvements in national health indicators have occurred to different degrees among LAC countries. Declining infant mortality rates are one of the most heralded successes of health improvements for the region over the last few decades. But if we take a closer look at the distribution of benefits, we find a pattern of improvement that translates into increasing gaps

[21] Almeida Filho N. Inequalities in health based on living conditions: Analysis of scientific output in Latin America and the Caribbean and annotated bibliography. Washington, DC: Pan American Health Organization; 1999. (Research in public health #19).

[22] Economic Commission for Latin America and the Caribbean. *Panorama Social de América Latina*. Santiago, Chile: ECLAC; 1998.

between the countries with higher and lower rates.

Specifically, infant mortality rates (IMR) declined more in absolute terms in countries with high initial rates, such as Bolivia and Haiti. But relative to the lowest IMR for the Region of the Americas, reductions were greater in countries with lower initial rates. There are only four countries in the Americas where the IMR fell by a factor of four or more between 1960–1964 and 1990–1994:

- Chile fell from 109 to 14, almost an eightfold reduction;
- Cuba fell from 59 to 10, almost a sixfold reduction;
- Costa Rica fell from 81 to 14, almost an eightfold reduction;
- Canada fell from 27 to 6, a 4.5-fold reduction.

Most of the countries with intermediate rates in the 1960–1964 period had reductions between 2.5 and 3.5 times in this 35-year period. During 1960–1964, ten countries had IMRs above 100. By the 1990–1994 period, three countries still claimed this dubious distinction, and the remaining six, excluding Chile, had reduced their rates only by factors of 2.5 or less. Although their initially high rate presented the potential for dramatic improvements similar to those seen in Canada, Chile, Cuba, and Costa Rica, these countries were not able to capitalize on this opportunity. The behavior of ratios between the infant mortality rates in each country and the minimum in the Americas during these periods is shown in Figure 2.

During 1960–1964, the IMR for the country with the highest rate was seven times higher than that for the country with the lowest rate in the Americas. But by 1990–1994, that ratio had risen to 14. The median value of these country ratios rose from 4 to 6 in the same period. The lower quartile rose from 2.5 to 3.3 and the upper quartile, from 4.8 to 8.0, so that the inter-quartile range increases from 2.3 to 4.7, more than doubling. The trend of the increasing inter-quartile range seems to have

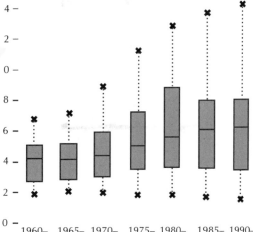

FIGURE 2.   Ratio between the value of infant mortality rate in each country and the minimum achieved in the Americas, 1960–1994.

slowed in the last two periods, and for some countries the ratios are beginning to decrease. But the median value continues to increase, and it is too early to predict if the improvements among the inter-quartile countries will continue, stabilize, or worsen.

The health disparities among countries in LAC become even more pronounced when comparing the ratio of national (estimated) maternal mortality rates with the minimum rate in the Region. While the IMR ratio between the countries with the highest and lowest rates is currently close to 14 in the Region, the ratios for maternal mortality are over 100 in two countries and over 20 in more than half of them. These enormous differences in maternal mortality possibly have much to do with inaccessibility to health care of acceptable quality. It is important to stress that a large proportion of infant deaths relates to environmentally related conditions—diarrheal disease, acute respiratory infections, malnutrition—whereas maternal mortality is almost wholly attributable to a lack of—or poor quality—prenatal, delivery, and puerperal care (see Figure 3).

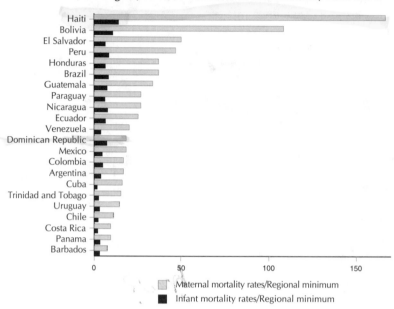

FIGURE 3. Ratio of the maternal mortality rate and the minimum achieved in the Region, compared with the ratio of the infant mortality rates and the minimum in the Region, selected countries in the Americas, circa 1994.

HEALTH INEQUALITIES WITHIN COUNTRIES

A general pattern of socioeconomic disparities in health among countries can be seen clearly within countries. The few studies of the relationships between socioeconomic conditions and health in LAC consistently find large health differentials between the upper and lower levels of well-being, be it measured by income, education level, spatial distributions, ethnicity, gender, access to health services, or national origin.

Income, Household Expenditure, or Other Material Living Conditions

Income is a useful socioeconomic category in the sense that it tends to be associated with a variety of other determinants, either for sociocultural reasons or for simple economics, depending on the particular population and social context studied. A few studies at the country level, within regions of countries, and at the local level have addressed disparities in health outcomes and access to care among populations with varied incomes. The health measures used range from the extreme of infant and childhood (ages 1–4 years) mortality, to low birthweight, stunting, and general childhood diseases.

Between 1982 and 1987, mortality between ages one and four was measured in southern Brazil for children in three economic categories: family incomes under US$ 50 per month (very low income), family incomes between US$ 50 and US$ 149 per month (low income), and family incomes above US$ 150 per month (see Figure 4). For very low income families the mortality rate for low birthweight children is almost six times higher than for children who were born weighing 3,000 g or more, but is practically the same when the family income is US$ 150 or more. And among all children born with normal birthweight (over 2,500 g), the mortality rate is five times higher in very

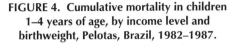

FIGURE 4. Cumulative mortality in children 1–4 years of age, by income level and birthweight, Pelotas, Brazil, 1982–1987.

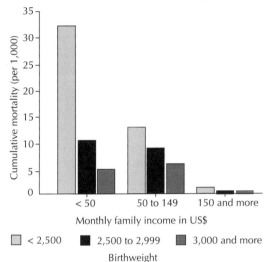

low income families when compared to families with incomes of US$ 150 and more.[23]

In a 1992 study in Barquisimeto, a medium-sized city in Venezuela, each of the 900 *barrios* (communities) was classified in terms of living conditions according to the accessibility of sanitation, adult literacy rate, and general condition of the dwellings. When comparing the 10% of the barrios with the worst living conditions with the 10% with the best living conditions, the incidence of low birthweight was almost twice as high for those with worse living conditions (almost 14% compared to 7%). The incidence of very low birthweight (under 1,500 g) was three times as high for those living in the worst conditions.[24]

Country studies of time trends indicate that relative levels of health disparities between socioeconomic groups are not changing. In a southern city in Brazil, children of two co-horts—born in 1982 and in 1993—presented

similar levels of disparities, in relative terms, between the lowest and highest income groups for almost all health indicators. Between 1982 and 1993, infant mortality for children of families with monthly incomes of one minimum wage or less decreased from 80 to 33 per 1,000 live births, while the rate in the highest income group of ten minimum wages or more dropped from 13 to 5 per 1,000 live births. Notwithstanding the overall improvement in IMR for all socioeconomic groups, the rate ratio between the low and high income brackets actually remained at the same level of 2.6 in that period of time.[25]

The prevalence of stunting in children younger than age 5 in Brazil in 1989 was roughly 30 times higher in families with per capita monthly incomes under US$ 20, when compared to families with per capita monthly incomes of US$ 160 or more, ranging from 28.9% to 0.9%. Another study in 1996 showed that households with no durable goods had a prevalence rate of 22.6%, compared to 4.4% for households with five or more durable goods. Similar results were also found in a cohort in southern Brazil, where the prevalence rate of stunting in households with only one durable good was 26%, compared to 7% for those with four or more such goods.[26]

The IMR in Peru for the poorest quintile is close to five times higher than that for the upper quintile. This ratio is close to seven for the mortality rate from 1 to 4 years of age. The prevalence of childhood diseases in Peru in 1996 according to the bottom and top quintiles of household assets varied between 25% and 15% for acute respiratory infections and between 22% and 13% for diarrhea (see Figure 5).[27]

[23] Victora C, Barros F, Hutley S, Teixeira AM, Vaughn JP. Early childhood mortality in a Brazilian cohort: The roles of bithweight and socioeconomic status. *Intern J Epidemiol* 1992; 21: 423–432.

[24] Montilva C. Universidad Central Occidental de Venezuela. (Personal communication).

[25] Victora C. Reducing health inequalities: Can health interventions make an impact? Paper presented at the Ninth Annual Public Health Forum. London: London School of Hygiene and Tropical Medicine; 1999.

[26] Olinto MTA, Victora CG, Barros FC and Tomasi E. Determinantes da desnutrição infantil em uma população de Baixa Renda: Um modelo de análise hierarquizado. *Cad Saúde Pública* 1993; 9 (Supl. 1): 14–27.

[27] World Bank. *Fact sheets on health, nutrition, population and poverty in Peru: Poverty thematic group.* Washington, DC: World Bank; 1999.

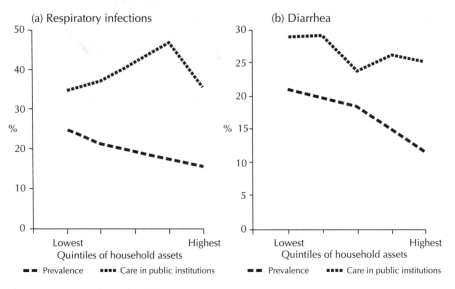

FIGURE 5. Prevalence of acute respiratory infections and diarrhea in children under 5 years of age, and treatment in public health institutions, Peru, 1996.

Source: Demographic and Health Survey, Peru, 1996.

In addition to a greater burden of disease, the poor also have less access to health services when they need care. Among those who were sick in the above study in Peru, proportionately more from the better-off quintiles sought care in public care facilities. Further, percentages of pregnant women who received prenatal care from trained personnel differed between the first and fifth quintiles of household assets, rising from 40% to 95%, while the figures for deliveries attended by trained personnel rose even more dramatically, from 15% to 96% (see Figure 6).[28]

Similar results were seen in Mexico in 1990–1996. The percentage of deliveries in hospitals increased from 8% in the municipalities in the lowest decile of average household income to 93% in the municipalities in the high-

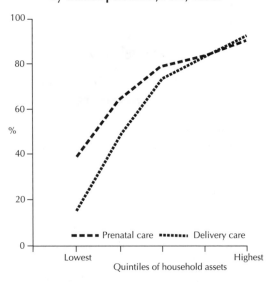

FIGURE 6. Percentage of pregnant women who received prenatal care and delivery by trained personnel, Peru, 1996.

Source: Demographic and Health Survey, Peru, 1996.

---

[28] World Bank. *Fact sheets on health, nutrition, population and poverty in Peru: Poverty thematic group.* Washington, DC: World Bank; 1999.

FIGURE 7. Distribution of health resources according to per capita income in municipalities, Mexico, 1990–1996.

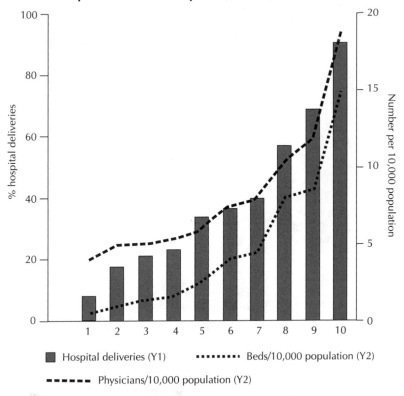

Hospital deliveries (Y1)   ▪▪▪▪▪▪▪▪ Beds/10,000 population (Y2)

▬ ▬ ▬ ▬ Physicians/10,000 population (Y2)

Source: Lozano R, Zurita B, Franco F, Ramírez T, Torres JL, Hernández P. Health inequality in Mexico: Study by socioeconomic strata at the country and household level. Preprint. Chapter of a book on the Global Health Equity Initiative to be published by the Rockefeller Foundation in 2000.

est decile of incomes. The number of hospital beds per 10,000 population varied from around 2 in the municipalities in the lowest decile of per capita income to 15 in the highest decile, and the percentage of deliveries in hospitals goes from less than 10% to over 90% in those same groups (see Figure 7).[29]

A recent study of the city of Rosario, Argentina indicated that poor women in greater need of services are not necessarily the ones who receive benefits, even when interventions are inexpensive and cost-effective. Women attended in public hospitals delivered babies with a mean neonatal weight of almost 200 g less than those delivering in the private clinics (3,168 grams and 3,350 g, respectively), and the still birth rate was 11.1 per 1,000 live births compared to 3.8 per 1,000. Yet, women delivering in public hospitals, most of whom had lower income levels, received iron and folic acid supplementation during the pregnancy in only 5.6% of cases, compared to 44.0% of cases for those delivering in private clinics. The percentages for other vitamin and mineral supplements were 0.3% and 24.8%, respectively, and for antibiotics, 4.8% and 15.7%, respectively.[30]

[29] Lozano R, Zurita B, Franco F, Ramírez T, Tores JL, Hernández P. Health inequality in Mexico: Study by socioeconomic strata at the country and household level. Preprint. Chapter of a book on the Global Health Equity Initiative to be published by the Rockefeller Foundation in 2000.

[30] Belizán JM, Farnot U, Carroll G, Al-Mazrou Y. Antenatal care in developing countries. *Paediatric and Perinatal Epidemiology* 1998; 12 (Suppl. 2) 1–3.

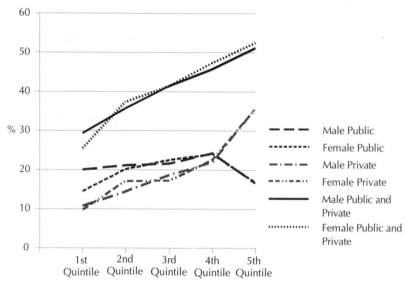

FIGURE 8. Median of the percentage of persons who sought health care among those who reported having some disease in the four weeks preceding the survey, by sex and by quintiles of per capita household consumption, according to the use of public and private services, selected countries in Latin America.

Source: Living Standards Measurement Surveys for Bolivia, Colombia, Ecuador, Nicaragua, and Venezuela, 1994–1996.

Little has been documented in terms of disparities in expenditure on health care in Latin American and Caribbean countries. An analysis of five countries, based on results of the LSMS surveys, indicates a gradient in the utilization of health care for persons with a *self-perceived need for care*, with higher utilization rates as family consumption increases. Although all groups present a similar rate of utilization of public services (around 20%), the lower income groups, as would be expected, have lower rates of utilization of private services (close to 10% in the lowest quintile) when compared to the higher groups (over 35% in the highest quintile) (see Figure 8).[31]

For those households where a health problem was declared to exist in the period previous to the survey, the average household health care expenditure in Nicaragua in 1993 represented almost 40% of total income for the

lowest quintile of income but less than 1% in the highest income quintile.[32] In the Dominican Republic, the poorest quintile paid 20% of their average household income on health care in 1996 while the highest quintile of income paid less than 10%.[33]

Level of Formal Education

In the area of formal education, there have been improvements in population coverage since 1985, but these advances have been smaller than in other regions of the world: by 1995, only two-thirds of the school-age population of Latin America and the Caribbean had completed the fourth year of basic education.

[31] Living Standards Measurement Studies for Bolivia, Ecuador, Colombia, Nicaragua, Venezuela, 1994–1996. See: *http://www.worldbank.org/html/prdph/lsml/lsmshome.html*

[32] Herrera J, Rivas W, Gadea A, Romero N, Bolaños L, Cáceres M, Campos F, Zamora JR. Cuentas nacionales en salud: Estudio de fuentes de financiamiento y gastos en salud 1995–1996. OPS/OMS, USAID, 1999.

[33] Rathe M. Cuentas nacionales de salud: Un análisis del financiamiento del sistema de salud de la República Dominicana. Santo Domingo, República Dominicana; 1998.

Southeast Asia, which had similar formal educational levels in 1985, has now surpassed LAC in the proportion of its population enrolled in primary and secondary education.[34] This finding may bode ill for improving health, given the proven correlation between family health and the formal education level of men and women. In response to the low development of formal education and its effect on opportunities and well being, the recent "Social Development Report" by the Inter-American Development Bank stressed the importance of increasing the access of poor children to formal education as the main intervention for poverty reduction and reducing inequalities in the Region.[35]

Specific studies have borne out these concerns. A national study in Brazil in 1996 showed that rates of stunting in children under 5 years old correspond strongly to the family's level of formal education. Rates range from 19.3% when the head of household has no formal education to only 3.4% when the family head has 11 or more years, an almost sixfold increase. Intermediate measures of formal education follow a corresponding pattern, with a 13.7% rate of stunting for 1 to 3 years of formal education, 8.0% for 4 to 7 years, and 6.3% for 8 to 10 years, indicating that any continuation of formal education may have a health impact. When the mother's formal educational level is analyzed, similar patterns emerge for both stunting—ranging from 19.9% for 0 to 3 years of formal education to 3.3% for 11 or more years—and for wasting—ranging from 24% for mothers with zero to three years of schooling to 7% when the mother has 6 or more years.[36]

Studies in Chile found relationships between women's formal education and their babies' health. Neonatal mortality rates stratified by maternal formal education level in Chile for the 1990–1995 period range from 13.5 per 1,000 live births for those with no formal education to 6 per 1,000 for those with 13 or more years. Post-neonatal mortality rates decline from 24.5 per 1,000 live births to 2.6 for the same categories, indicating a tenfold difference when the mother is illiterate as compared to mothers with 13 or more years of schooling (see Figure 9).[37]

A dramatic example that demonstrates the need to determine how benefits are being captured by socioeconomic groups is illustrated by the rise in life expectancy among Chilean women between the mid 1980s and the mid 1990s. Women in Chile gained almost two years in their life expectancy at age 20, but women with 13 years of formal education or more enjoyed almost all the benefits, gaining almost ten years in a ten-year period, while gains in the groups with lesser formal education levels were negligible (see Figure 10).[38]

Spatial Distributions

Studies show that health varies according to spatial distributions within countries, which have been measured between geographic regions, between urban and rural populations, and between wealthier and poorer communities. Data from the Demographic and Health Surveys (DHS) show, for example, how different the rates of stunting for children below 5 years of age are between urban and rural areas of various countries. In some cases, the percentage of children under the standard in rural areas is two-and-a-half times higher than in urban areas (Table 1).

In Peru and Guatemala, the prevalence of stunting in rural areas exceeds 50% of all chil-

[34] World Bank. *World Development Report 1998*. Washington, DC: World Bank; 1998.

[35] Inter-American Development Bank. *Economic and social progress in Latin America, 1998–1999 report: Facing up to inequality in Latin America*. Washington, DC: IADB; 1999.

[36] Epidemiological Studies in Health and Nutrition, Univeity of São Paulo. Melhoria em indicadores de saúde associados à pobreza no Brasil do sanos 90. University of São Paulo: School of Public Health. (Internal report).

[37] Hollstein RD, Vega JM, Carvajal YB. Socioeconomic level and infant mortality in Chile in the period 1985–1995. *Rev Med Chile* 1998; 126:333–340.

[38] Vega J, Holstein RD, Delgado I, Marshall G, Yach D. Social inequalities and health in an intermediate-development nation: Education and adult mortality in Chile, 1980–1996. Preprint. Chapter of a book on the Global Health Equity Initiative to be published by the Rockefeller Foundation in 2000.

FIGURE 9. Neonatal and post-neonatal mortality, Chile, 1990–1995.

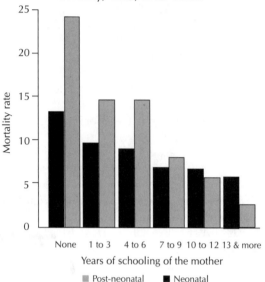

Years of schooling of the mother

■ Post-neonatal   ■ Neonatal

FIGURE 10. Life expectancy at age 20 according to years of schooling, females, Chile, 1985–1987 to 1994–1996.

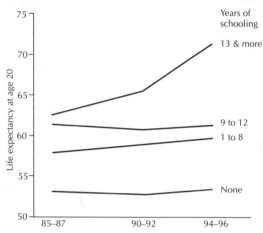

Source: Vega J, Hollstein RD, Delgado I, Marshall G, Yach D. Social inequities and health in an intermediate-development nation: Education and adult mortality in Chile, 1980–1996. Preprint. Chapter of a book on the Global Health Equity Initiative to be published by the Rockefeller Foundation in 2000.

dren below age 5.[39] In the city of Buenos Aires, Argentina, the IMR in 1995 was close to 13 per 1,000 live births, but some of the country's provinces have rates that exceed 30 per 1,000 live births.[40] In Chile, the years of potential life lost below age 65 in the *comunas* (counties) with better living conditions is close to 72 years per 1,000 population, but reaches almost 157 per 1,000 population in those with the worst living conditions.[41] In Mexico, the years of potential life lost below age 70 ranges from 10 to 181 per 1,000 population in municipalities with the lowest and highest values according to a deprivation index.[42]

[39] Macro International. Demographic and Health Surveys. Calverton, Maryland; 1996.
[40] Pan American Health Organization. *Health in the Americas, 1998 edition.*Washington, DC; PAHO; 1998.
[41] Concha M, Aguilera X, Guerrero A, Salas J, Child V. *Metodologías de apoyo a la priorización local de problemas de salud.* Santiago, Chile: Ministerio de Salud; 1997.
[42] Lozano R, Zurita B, Franco F, Ramírez T, Torres JL, Hernández P. Health inequality in Mexico: Study by socioeconomic strata at the country and household level. Preprint. Chapter of a book on the Global Health Equity Initiative to be published by the Rockefeller Foundation in 2000.

Infant mortality in Brazil fell 40% between 1977–1985 and 1987–1995, but the gaps between the worse-off areas, with high rates, and the ones with lowest rates have increased. Table 2 presents the rates estimated from data of Demographic and Health Surveys of 1986 and 1996 by the five great geographical regions for rural and urban areas of Brazil. The mortality rates fell in all areas, but the rate ratios of the worst part (north-east-rural) and the whole country increased from 1.7 to 2.0. Stunting below age five fell in Northeastern

TABLE 1. Percentage of stunting in children under 5 years of age, by urban or rural area, selected countries in Latin America and the Caribbean, early to mid 1990s.

Country and year	Urban (%)	Rural (%)
Dominican Republic, 1996	7.3	15.2
Brazil, 1996	7.8	19.0
Colombia, 1995	12.5	19.1
Paraguay, 1990	11.7	26.9
Haiti, 1995	20.4	35.1
Bolivia, 1994	20.9	36.6
Peru, 1992	25.9	53.4
Guatemala, 1995	35.3	56.6

TABLE 2. Trends in infant mortality rates, by geographical region and urban/rural strata, Brazil, 1977–1985 and 1987–1995.

Stratum/region	1977–1985	1987–1995	Annual change (%)
Urban	68.8	41.2	– 4.0
North	(51.1)	(42.1)	– 1.7
Northeast	120.4	62.8	– 4.8
South-Central	47.0	33.0	– 3.0
Rural[a]	100.9	60.8	– 4.0
Northeast	135.2	84.4	– 3.7
South-Central	(61.2)	28.8	– 5.3
Brazil[b]	79.6	46.1	– 4.2

Source: Pan American Health Organization, Division of Health and Human Development (DHS), 1986, 1996.

[a]Rates based on less than 1,000.

[b]Does not include the rural areas of the Northern region.

Brazil from 47.8% in 1975, to 27.3% in 1989, and to 17.9% in 1996. In the South-Central region the prevalence declined from 23.9% to 8.6% to 5.6% in the same years. In 21 years, the prevalence fell almost fourfold in the better-off regions but only 2.7-fold in the worst one. The rate ratios were 2.0 in 1975, and over 5 in 1996.[43]

Ethnicity

Two ethnic groups in LAC are generally recognized as particularly vulnerable populations—the indigenous population and the population of African descent. Studies by the Inter-American Development Bank point out that there are approximately 150 million persons of African descent in Latin America. Of all the poor in Latin America, 40% are of African descent.[44] Preliminary health data from Colombia's Pacific coast and evidence elsewhere suggest that Black communities suffer poor health disproportionately.[45] Racial categories for populations in the Americas correlate with other socioeconomic indicators, such as income, education, and geography.

Since the 1990s, some countries in the Region have made significant efforts to collect and analyze statistics based on race and ethnicity. Belize, Bolivia, Brazil, Ecuador, Chile, Guatemala, El Salvador, Mexico, Nicaragua, Paraguay, and Peru already include the variable of ethnicity in their national statistics. In other cases, the stratification of data by geographic location (urban vs. rural vs. hinterland or by ethnically homogeneous small areas) is a proxy method for identifying significant disparities in the health situation between ethnic groups.

It also is necessary to recognize the differences in concepts and application of race and ethnicity in North America, Latin America, and the Caribbean and to see them as the social constructs that they are. Historical and cultural factors account for the fact that race underscores a phenotype that differentiates human beings by skin color, whereas ethnic groups display cultural characteristics beyond skin color. In any case, the countries' historical and cultural development, as well as the level of relative empowerment of different ethnic groups, will determine the categories of analysis which need to be studied and monitored in every particular case.

The results of the relatively few studies of socioeconomic conditions of Latin America's indigenous populations are instructive.[46] They

[43] Epidemiological Studies in Health and Nutrition, University of São Paulo. Melhoria em indicadores de saúde associados à pobreza no Brasil dos anos 90. University of São Paulo: School of Public Health. (Internal report).

[44] These data do not include the Dominican Republic and Cuba.

[45] Cowater International Inc., Inter-American Development Bank. Poverty alleviation for communities of African ancestry. Washington, DC; 1996.

[46] World Bank, Technical Division, Latin American and Caribbean Division. *Indigenous people and poverty in Latin America: An empirical analysis.* Washington, DC: World Bank; 1993.

confirm that the level of poverty among indigenous people in LAC is very high.

- In Bolivia over two-thirds of the bilingual indigenous population and almost three-fourths of the non-bilingual population are poor.
- In Guatemala, the majority of the indigenous population does not have access to such public services as water, sanitation, and electricity, and approximately half of the indigenous households have no access to safe water and basic sanitary services compared with 5% of the non-indigenous population.
- In Bolivia formal education levels of the indigenous population are three years less, on average, than the non-indigenous population.
- In Mexico poverty is highly correlated to municipalities with indigenous populations.
- Recent poverty studies in LAC communities with African ancestry identified similar trends. Poverty in these communities ranges from as low as 2% in the populations of Bolivia and Costa Rica to as high as 40% to 50% in Brazil and Colombia.[47]

As expected, patterns of health outcomes according to race or ethnicity follow these patterns of socioeconomic conditions. The few studies on the topic that have been published confirm large disparities between the health of indigenous groups and national statistics:

- For indigenous groups in the Region, infant mortality is 3.5 times higher in Panama, life expectancy is 29 years lower for men and 27 years lower for women in Honduras, child mortality is more than 2.5 times higher in Mexico, and maternal mortality is 83% higher in Guatemala.[48]
- A 1993/1994 survey in Colombia of 11,522 Native Americans living in indigenous com-

munities located in three geographically and culturally distinct communities—the Caribbean, the Amazon Basin, and the Andes—found that health indicators among those populations were significantly worse than for most Colombians. Life expectancy at birth for indigenous populations in 1993 was 57.8 years for women and 55.4 years for men, compared to national averages of 67 and 65 years. The infant mortality rate for these populations in 1990 was 63.3 per 1,000 live births, compared to the national average of 32.[49]

- Again, these populations tend to have disproportionately low levels of access to care. In Bolivia, indigenous people report more than twice the number of illnesses and injuries and are off from work twice the number of days. However, they receive less medical help or care and have access to less preventive care such as vaccination for yellow fever than the Mestizo population, which composes the majority of the national population.
- Government efforts in Guatemala have expanded the coverage of immunization programs in rural areas, but the data shows that percentage of children without access to any form of immunization, or restricted access to health services, information, and health promotion is still higher among indigenous and rural communities (see Figures 11, 12, and 13).[50]
- A 1990 study in Brazil addresses infant mortality in relation to both race and maternal formal education, and shows that for illiterate mothers IMRs were close to 120 per

---

[47] Cowate A International Inc., Inter-American Development Bank. Poverty alleviation for communities of African ancestry. Washington, DC; 1996.

[48] Amaris A, Flores C, Mojica J. Mortalidad infantil en Panamá: Un análisis de sus tendencias derivadas del censo 1990. Panamá; 1992. Rivas R. Pueblos indígenas y

Garífunas. Honduras: Guaymuras; 1993. Instituto Nacional Indigenista. La salud de los pueblos indígenas en México. México, DF: Secretaría de Salud; 1993. Health of indigenous peoples. *Rev Panam Salud Publica.*

[49] Piñeros-Petersen M, Ruiz-Salguero M. Aspectos demográficos en comunidades indígenas de tres regiones de Colombia. *Salud Publica Mex* 1998: Jul–Aug; 40(4):324–329. United Nations. *World population prospects, 1998 revision.* New York, NY: UN; 1998. Pan American Health Organization. *Health statistics from the Americas, 1998 edition.* Washington, DC: PAHO; 1998.

[50] Pan American Health Organization, Health and Human Development, Public Policy and Health Program. Health systems inequalities and poverty in Latin America and the Caribbean: Trends and policy implications. Washington, DC: PAHO. (EquiLac/IHEP draft document); 1999.

FIGURE 11. Gaps in delivery care: place of birthing by ethnic group and area of residence, Guatemala, 1995.

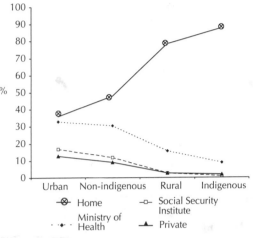

Source: INE (1996a).

FIGURE 13. Percentage of women of child-bearing age who knew about AIDS and percentage of those who knew about protection methods, Guatemala, 1995.

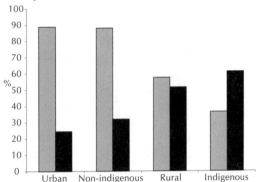

Source: INE (1996a).

1,000 for blacks, 110 for mulattos and dark-skinned, and 95 for whites. For mothers with eight or more years of formal education, the rates were much lower, respectively 82, 70, and 57 per 1,000 live births, but these rates presented even greater relative disparities according to race than they did to formal education (see Figure 14). Black women needed between four and seven years of formal education before they could achieve the IMRs of illiterate white women,

FIGURE 12. Gaps in immunization: percentage of children with complete immunization and with no immunization, by area of residence and ethnicity, Guatemala, 1995.

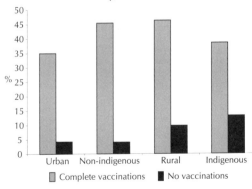

Source: INE (1996a).

demonstrating the strength of the effect of ethnically based discrimination in health.[51]

Gender

In addition to the differences in health needs that are biologically derived and specific to each sex, there are gender inequalities in health outcomes, access to care, utilization and financing of services that are socially produced. These gender inequalities constitute a reflection of the differences in women's and men's social roles, and of their relative positioning in terms of access to resources and power over health determinants.

An illustrative example of the interaction of gender and socioeconomic inequities is contained in Table 3 and in Figures 15 and 16, which show the probability of dying between 15 to 59 years of age for poor and non-poor males and females in 13 countries of the Region.[52] The generally recognized fact that

[51] Pinto da Cunha E. Raça: Aspecto esquecido da inequidade em saúde no Brasil. In Barata R et al.: *Equidade e saúde: Contribuições da epidemiologia*. Rio de Janeiro, Brazil: Abrasco/Fio Cruz; 1997.

[52] World Health Organization. *The World Health Report, 1999*. Geneva: WHO; 2000.

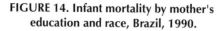

FIGURE 14. Infant mortality by mother's education and race, Brazil, 1990.

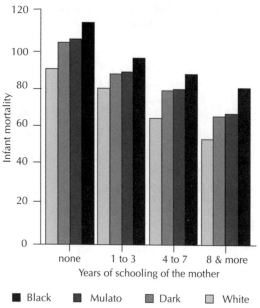

Hostile conditions in the social environment and lack of appropriate health services seem to disproportionately affect women's opportunities for health and health care, curtailing—or in some rare instances, eliminating—the long-standing biological advantage of female survival.

The fact that women live longer does not mean that they need less health care. On the contrary, women's need for health services is greater than that of men, due primarily to the female reproductive function. Women also tend to exhibit higher rates of morbidity throughout their lives and because of their greater longevity they additionally bear a heavier burden of chronic disease. In fact, in every country and at every socioeconomic level, women consistently report a higher incidence of health problems. Even though women tend to utilize health services more often than men, if utilization is measured in relation to expressed need for care, women actually are less likely to utilize health services than men, particularly among the poor (see Figure 8).

mortality rates are higher among males at any age is clearly depicted by the higher male/female risk ratio of premature death—which varies from 1.6 to 4.0 among the non-poor. Among the poor, however, this ratio is considerably reduced and even reversed in some countries. In other words, poverty does not appear to be an equal opportunity dispenser of premature death among men and women.

LSMS data from Peru corroborates the overall higher frequency with which women report health problems (disease and accidents) and utilize health services (see Table 4 and Figure 17). Indeed, women report 15% more health problems than men. However, when it comes to receiving health care, their use of

TABLE 3. Probability of dying (per 100) between 15 to 59 years of age, by income and sex, 13 Latin American and Caribbean countries.

Country	Male poor	Female poor	Male non-poor	Female non-poor	Poor male/female ratio	Non-poor male/female ratio
Brazil	'55.2	47.4	23	6	1.2	3.8
Chile	44.4	36.9	12	3	1.2	4.0
Colombia	52.5	52	25	10	1.0	2.5
Costa Rica	38.5	31.8	7	3	1.2	2.3
Dominican Republic	40.8	48.5	12	5	0.8	2.4
Ecuador	48.6	48.4	18	11	1.0	1.6
Guatemala	43.7	31.4	23	9	1.4	2.6
Honduras	30	28	15	7	1.1	2.1
Mexico	46.4	43	16	5	1.1	3.2
Nicaragua	33.6	33.6	16	6	1	2.7
Panama	33.3	30.8	9	4	1.1	2.3
Peru	27.2	21.6	16	6	1.3	2.7
Venezuela	48	45.6	16	6	1.1	2.7

Source: World Health Organization. *The World Health Report, 1999.* Geneva: WHO; 2000.

FIGURE 15. Probability of premature mortality (per 100),
15–59 years of age, by sex and level of poverty,
13 Latin American and Caribbean countries, 1994.

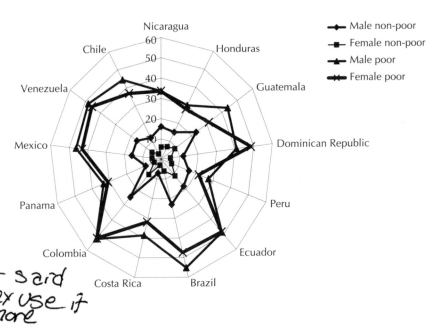

*Just said
they use it
more*

health services is only 2% higher than that of men. Furthermore, the tendency toward higher utilization of female services completely vanishes in the lowest income quintile where, paradoxically, the gender gap in health-need is widest. Thus, despite the oft-

noted higher utilization of services by women, this pattern is still far from approaching the equity principle of securing access to services according to need.

Finally, because of their greater need for health care and the features of current financial systems, women have higher out-of-pocket expenses, both in absolute terms as well as in relation to their income or their to-

FIGURE 16. Poor/non-poor ratio in the probability of dying (per 100) between 15 and 59 years of age, by sex, 13 Latin American and Caribbean countries.

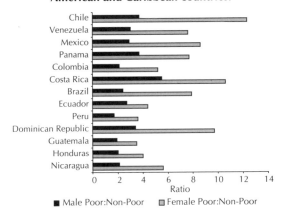

TABLE 4. Percent difference between females and males in perception of health problems and utilization of health services, by income quintiles, Peru, 1997.

Income quintiles	Perception of health problems (females/males × 100)	Utilization of services (females/males ×100)
Total	14.7	2.2
I (Low)	16.5	–0.5
II	12.4	2
III	14.8	2.2
IV	15.8	4.5
V (High)	13.4	5.3

Source: Living Standards Measurement Study (LSMS) survey, Peru, 1997.

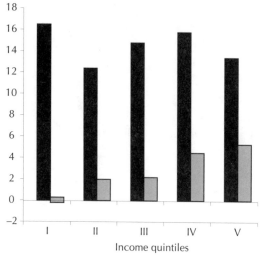

FIGURE 17. Peru: percent difference between females and males in perception of health problems and utilization of health services, by income quintiles, 1997.

Income quintiles

■ Perception of health problems (females/males × 100)
☐ Utilization of services (females/males × 100)

Source: Living Standards Measurement Study, Peru 1997.

tal household expenditures. This higher expenditure has implications not only for women's health but also for their financial well-being. Survey data recently reviewed in PAHO's Division of Health and Human Development for four countries show that women's out-of-pocket expenditures for health care ranged between 15% to over 40% higher than men's (see Table 5). This disparity in expenditure is compounded by the fact that throughout the Region women's income remains below that of men. For example, in 16 countries of the Americas, women's earnings in urban areas continue to range from under 60% to less than 80% of men's average income.[53] Furthermore, to the extent that health care and social security financing are dependent on employment status, gender disparities in access to services will continue to exist due to women's disadvantaged position in the labor market. This disadvantage derives from the social centrality of reproduction in women's lives which keeps more than 50% of females outside the paid labor market, concentrates those who are employed in occupations that are poorly remunerated or fall outside the coverage of social benefits—such as part-time or informal-sector jobs—and introduces discontinuity in their work histories.

Physical and Financial Access to Health Services

A series of case studies on health system inequalities was undertaken within the framework of a joint PAHO/UNDP/World Bank Project on Investment in Health, Equity, and Poverty in Latin America and the Caribbean (EquiLac/IHEP). The countries under investigation—Brazil, Ecuador, Guatemala, Jamaica, Mexico, and Peru—account for more than two-thirds of the population, Gross Domestic Product (GDP), and overall national health expenditure of the 45 countries and territories in Latin America and the Caribbean. Among the fundamental issues addressed were (a) the extent to which differences in organization, delivery, and financing of national health care systems are relevant in explaining health systems inequalities, and (b) the response of different national systems to the needs of the poor.[54]

The population of the countries ranges from 3 million in the case of Jamaica to 94 million in Mexico and 163 million in Brazil. Differences in per capita income in these countries, expressed in US$ adjusted for purchasing power parity (PPP), range from close to US$ 4,000 in Guatemala to around US$ 6,300 in Brazil and US$ 7,600 in Mexico. Brazil and Guatemala are the countries with the greatest degree of income inequality; the Gini coefficient for these two countries is around 0.60,

[53] Economic Commission for Latin America and the Caribbean. *Panorama social de America Latina.* Santiago, Chile: ECLAC; 1998.

[54] Pan American Health Organization, Health and Human Development, Public Policy and Health Program. Health systems inequalities and poverty in Latin America and the Caribbean: Trends and policy implications. Washington, DC: PAHO. (EquiLac/IHEP draft document); 1999.

TABLE 5. Out-of-pocket expenditures for health, by gender, selected Latin American and Caribbean countries.

Country	Health spending (current US$)		Health expenditures as a percent of total household spending	
	Data	Percent difference	Data	Percent difference
Brazil				
Females	$239.51	**40.0**	2.1	**40.0**
Males	$171.08		1.5	
Paraguay				
Females	$381.95	**27.4**	4.5	**28.6**
Males	$299.77		3.5	
Peru				
Females	$100.31	**41.5**	2.0	**42.9**
Males	$70.91		1.4	
Dominican Republic				
Females	$162.52	**14.9**	8.5	**14.9**
Males	$141.48		7.4	

Source: Living Standards Measurement Study surveys for Brazil, Paraguay, and Peru; Demographic and Health Surveys for the Dominican Republic.

while the ratio of the share of income going to the top and bottom quintiles of the income distribution is 47 in Brazil and 32 in Guatemala. Jamaica has the lowest level of income inequality, with a Gini coefficient of 41 and an income share ratio of top to bottom quintiles of 8. The population living below a consumption-based poverty line—defined as those whose income is below the cost of a market basket of commodities providing a minimum intake or consumption of calories and proteins—ranges from more than 50% in Ecuador, Peru, and Guatemala to 34% in Jamaica, 17% in Brazil, and 10% in Mexico. In Jamaica, 34% of the population has an income below the poverty line (see Table 6).

The national health systems of these countries range from predominantly public, as is the case of Jamaica and Mexico, to a wide variety of mixed systems, as are the cases of Brazil, Ecuador, and Peru. In all countries, private expenditures, including direct out-of-pocket expenditures and voluntary contributions to privately managed prepaid health plans and health insurance schemes, are the largest component of national health care expenditures, ranging from 66% in Brazil to around 50% in Ecuador, Jamaica, and Peru. For developed countries excluding the US, the public-private mix is around 70/30. There are even wider variations in out-of-pocket expenditure. It is 40% in Brazil, while in Ecuador and Peru, where only 20% of the population is covered by national health insurance, direct out-of-pocket sources is the main component of financing national health expenditure, a

TABLE 6. Selected indicators for countries participating in the EquiLAC and IHEP projects.

Country	Population (millions)	Per capita income PPP (US$)	Gini coefficient	Ratio 20/20	Population below PL-C[a] (%)
Brazil	165.2	6,340	60	32	27.2
Ecuador	12.2	4,730	47	20	54.7
Guatemala[a]	11.6	3,820	50	31	75.2
Jamaica	2.5	3,450	41	8	34.2
Mexico	95.8	7,660	50	14	38.6
Peru	24.7	4,410	45	12	49.0

Source: World Bank, SID-CG, PAHO Health Status Indicators, 1999.
[a]PL-C: Poverty line, consumption-based.

TABLE 7. Distribution of Ministry of Health subsidy, by income quintiles, urban and rural areas, and type of establishment, Peru, 1997.

| | Percentages | | | | Cumulative percentages | | | |
| | URBAN | | RURAL | | URBAN | | RURAL | |
Quintile	Hospitals	Health centers/ posts MINSA	Hospitals	Health centers/ posts MINSA	Hospitals	Health centers/ posts MINSA	Hospitals	Health centers/ posts MINSA
1 (Low)	18.1	24.3	6.0	17.8	18.1	24.3	6.0	17.8
2	20.5	22.5	10.4	16.6	38.6	46.8	16.5	34.4
3	19.7	21.5	19.2	25.1	58.3	68.4	35.7	59.5
4	21.1	21.0	31.9	17.5	79.5	89.3	67.6	76.9
5 (High)	20.5	10.7	32.4	23.1	100.0	100.0	100.0	100.0

situation which is evidently discriminatory and greatly affects the ability of the poor and disadvantaged in the Region to obtain needed health care.

One example of the disparities that exist in the use of public resources is contained in Table 7, which presents the distribution of the subsidies provided by the Ministry of Health of Peru, according to income quintiles, for urban and rural areas and by type of establishment. The results show that with the exception of Health Centers and Posts, for which the subsidies are more concentrated in the lower quintiles (poorest households), the distribution is uniform at best (i.e., approximately the same for all income groups) as in the case of urban hospitals, or very skewed in favor of the rich as in the case of rural hospitals. Within rural hospitals, almost two-thirds of the resources are used by households in the two upper income quintiles.

The same data from Peru are also presented in several concentration curves (see Figure 18). For the curves corresponding to urban hospitals and to rural health centers/posts, the distribution is almost equal. The urban health centers/posts present a progressive distribution. Rural hospitals, on the other hand, evince an extremely regressive distribution, favoring the rich.

Using a methodology for measuring inequalities in health status and in the delivery of health care that was originally developed

for a project in ten European Union countries,[55] the study concluded that, despite the diversity of socioeconomic conditions and a variety of organizational, financing, and delivery systems, some common patterns emerged:

• Whereas the differences in perceived health status as measured by self-reported symptoms of illness or accident and self-assessed health between the various income groups are relatively small, differences in health status as measured by the incidence and prevalence of diseases and mortality are quite large. The low income groups are more exposed to environmental risks, are more frequently sick, live shorter lives, and report more days of lost work due to illness and disability.
• The size of the gap between health needs and utilization of health services is inversely correlated to the level of income. The lower the level of income, the larger the gap between health needs and utilization of health services.
• Distribution of private consumption expenditures compounds the socioeconomic differences associated with income/expenditure distribution.
• The larger the share of government expenditure as a percentage of national health care

[55] Van Doorslaer E, Wagstaff A, Rutter F (eds). *Equity in the finance and delivery of health care.* New York, NY: Oxford University Press; 1993.

FIGURE 18. Concentration curves for the distribution of the Ministry of Health subsidies by type of establishment (hospital or health center, and urban or rural area) and by income quintiles, Peru, 1997 (Living Standards Measurement Study survey data).

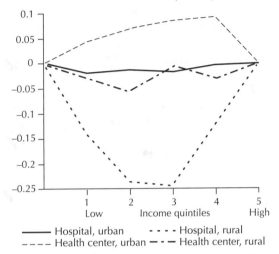

Legend:
——— Hospital, urban   · · · · Hospital, rural
– – – Health center, urban — · — Health center, rural

Source: EquiLAC project report, PAHO, Health in Human Development, 1999.

expenditure, the lower the differences in health care service utilization and the differences between overall consumption expenditures between high and low income groups.

- The distributive impact of government expenditures in health care services is limited by the relatively low utilization of health care services by the poor.

Based on the results from the case studies, the report made the following observations and suggestions related to the development of policy.

- The lack of significant differences in the perception of symptoms of illness or accidents among income groups suggests that the service availability may not be a major constraint on access for the poor, but rather that differing thresholds of self-perceived health and disease and other cultural, economic, and social barriers may be of more

importance in explaining disparities in health service utilization.

- Increasing availability of health care services may not result in an increase in the utilization of these services even if the services are provided free of charge or for a nominal fee. It is necessary to increase awareness among the lower income groups and the uneducated about their real need for health care, and to encourage and assist the poor to make fuller use of health care facilities for preventive purposes.

- Greater emphasis should be placed on evaluating the determinants of health status of different socioeconomic groups so as to provide a better understanding of the relevant types of health policies and health care services required to break the cycle of poverty. Improving equity in access to supply driven interventions (mainly preventative and health promotion activities, as well as health information) may improve overall population health more than demand driven services, which are more aligned to providing individual satisfaction of a perceived need.

- The development of more sensitive and specific measurements of health status, health service access and utilization, and health needs are required in order to better explore the determinants and interactions between health disparities and access to health services among the particular population subgroups. Also, there is a need to link traditional epidemiological methods and data sources (vital registries, disease surveillance, health service production statistics) with emerging sources of reliable useful data on living conditions, health status, and health service utilization, such as periodic national household surveys for monitoring of demographic, social, and economic trends (LSMS, DHS, MECOVI[56]). PAHO,

---

[56] MECOVI: "Mejoramiento de Encuestas de Condiciones de Vida" is a UNDP, IADB, WB, ECLAC, and PAHO initiative to improve design and utilization of household surveys for use by a broader range of economic and social sector monitoring and planning purposes, including health.

through the Division of Health and Human Development's Public Policy and Health Program, is to become the fourth member institution of the MECOVI Project, which is working to improve the health component of the instruments used in the surveys, and the use of the data to study inequalities in health status, access, utilization and financing of health care. As part of this effort, a database of existing surveys is now available online with information on almost 100 surveys used in the past 15 years that have a health module, including all countries in Latin America and several in the Caribbean.

Health, National Origin, and Migration

The relationship between health and internal and international migration has been recognized for many years. The effects of migration can be observed both in the place of origin as well as at the destination, and affect health status, access to health care, and demand for health services. In general, migrant populations have worse health status and less access to health services than non-migrants. Taking this into consideration, the World Health Organization (WHO) and the International Organization for Migration (IOM) signed a Memorandum of Understanding in Geneva in October of 1999 to strengthen collaboration between the two organizations to "better meet the health needs of migrants and other displaced persons." Specific goals include to reduce the mortality, morbidity, and disability among migrants; to provide them with better health services; and to campaign for effective international health policies and support infrastructure for migrants.

International migration has increased considerably, and it is expected that this trend will continue. The most recent worldwide estimates of the number of international migrants (UNFPA) indicated that there were 120 million international migrants in 1990, accounting for about 2% of the world's population. At that time, the Region's countries that experienced significant effects from international immigration were the United States, Canada, Belize, Costa Rica, Argentina, Venezuela, Antigua and Barbuda, Bahamas, Barbados, and Saint Kitts and Nevis: the immigrants represent more than 5% of the total population in those countries.

From the perspective of the receiving countries and the immigration policies, IOM has defined six different types of international migrants: "permanent settlers," "documented labor migrants" (including both "temporary contract workers" and "temporary professional transients"), "undocumented migrants," "asylum seekers," "recognized refugees," and "*de facto* refugees" or "externally displaced persons." The respective health needs of these groups as well as the effect of their health status on the health services of the recipient countries is different for every type of migrant. This issue is being addressed in a study that Division of Health and Human Development's Public Policy and Health Program and PAHO's Country Office in Costa Rica are developing in that country at the request of the national authorities and USAID.[57]

COMMENTS AND DISCUSSION

Most countries in the Americas are currently undergoing health sector reforms. Often, these processes occur as part of broader State reforms intended to facilitate the integration of regional economies into the global market. Considering the enormous disparities in the socioeconomic status of the populations in this Region's countries, if these reforms are to succeed, they must take these inequalities into account. In terms of health, the reforms' main objective has to be coupled with general policies that diminish the gaps between the extremes of the socioeconomic spectrum and promote greater access to basic health care.

---

[57] Pan American Health Organization, Division of Health and Human Development, Public Policy and Health Program. Project document: Spatial mobility, processes of integration and health in Central America. Washington, DC: PAHO; 1999. (Mim. September 1999).

The Pan American Health Organization is promoting several studies and projects in this area, including a multicenter study in five countries, using data from LSMS and DHS surveys and from national censuses, to increase available knowledge about the inequalities in health and their relationships with many of their determinants. These studies emphasize the need for results that can be used to address policy issues and to design and evaluate interventions both within and outside of the health sector and to address these disparities in a meaningful way. The specific areas of actions required will vary from country to country, but the multiple causes of ill-health call for the following four levels of policy action: strengthening individuals, strengthening communities, improving access to basic services and facilities, and encouraging macroeconomic and cultural changes. Acting on these levels requires a strategic approach that takes into account the interrelationships across sectors and policy levels.[58]

Research provides crucial support to an equity-oriented policy agenda by providing data and analyses that address gaps in knowledge. In so doing, it helps to identify policy options and strategies, including those that would help redress power imbalances in the decision making process. The empowerment of the weak, the disadvantaged, and the marginalized requires increasing their access to information. In the words of Julio Frenk:

> If the evidence is clear and recommendations are vigorous, those who have the power to decide may be stimulated into action. At the very least, sound policy analysis places limits on the discretion of decision makers, who have to consider the costs of ignoring the available data.[59]

Given the strength of available evidence, it can be safely concluded that in LAC, as has been demonstrated in North America and Europe, the main social determinants of health are those related to differential power relations and opportunities, mainly evidenced by differences due to race or ethnicity, gender, and social class (as measured by income level, material living conditions, educational attainment, or occupation). A growing body of research has begun to develop alternative approaches to studying the health effects of these features, and these new inquiries are seeking to address the many limitations of the predominant epidemiological methods.[60] This work can be characterized by three basic assumptions about the nature of health and disease in human societies:

- Societal divisions based on race, gender, and class are the expression of social relations, not intrinsic facts of biology. Consequently, social factors, not genetics, primarily explain why people's membership in the groups defined by these social relations can predict their overall health status.
- The fact that population patterns of health and disease parallel societal divisions based on race, gender, and class implies that these relations somehow shape the health of groups on both sides of these social relations; disparate social and economic situations somehow become "incorporated" into biological pathways that affect health and survival.
- The responsible mechanisms exist at both the social and biological level, and both levels must be studied to understand what creates population patterns of health and disease.

Although the results of these studies point to large, persistent, and often increasing disparities in the Region, much more methodological and empirical research must be done to better study how and why socioeconomic factors are related to health status, access to

[58] Gilson L. In defence and pursuit of equity. Soc Sci Med 1998; 47: 1891–1896.

[59] Frenk, J. in Gilson L. In defence and pursuit of equity. Soc Sci Med 1998; 47: 1891–1896.

[60] Krieger N, Rowley DL, Herman AA, Avery B, Phillips MT. Racism, sexism and social class: Implications for studies of health, disease and well-being. Amer J Prevent Med 1993; 5 (suppl.).

FIGURE 19. Policy factors and mechanisms influencing personal and household health and welfare.

```
                    Political Systems and Processes
         Affects acceptance of discrimination, definition of public needs,
           determinants of public policy, level of civil society participation,
                accountability/transparency of public administration


                          Policies affecting
    Macro-economic           key assets
       Policy                                      Public provisioning
    Fiscal, monetary,    Labor policy, land distribution,        policy
   balance of payments,        housing policy          Education, social welfare, health
      trade policy                                      care, water and sanitation


    Patterns of        Employment levels        Migration patterns,
    investments,        and patterns,            remittance of
    price levels        demand for goods             income
                        and services


    Income/wealth levels/distribution, Food intake, Access to health promoting inputs
          Access to cost-effective quality health care and social services
                        Overall spatial development


                  Personal & Household Health and Welfare
        Quality of environment, disposable income, food production, health seeking behavior,
            household health investment, domestic allocation of time and resources
```

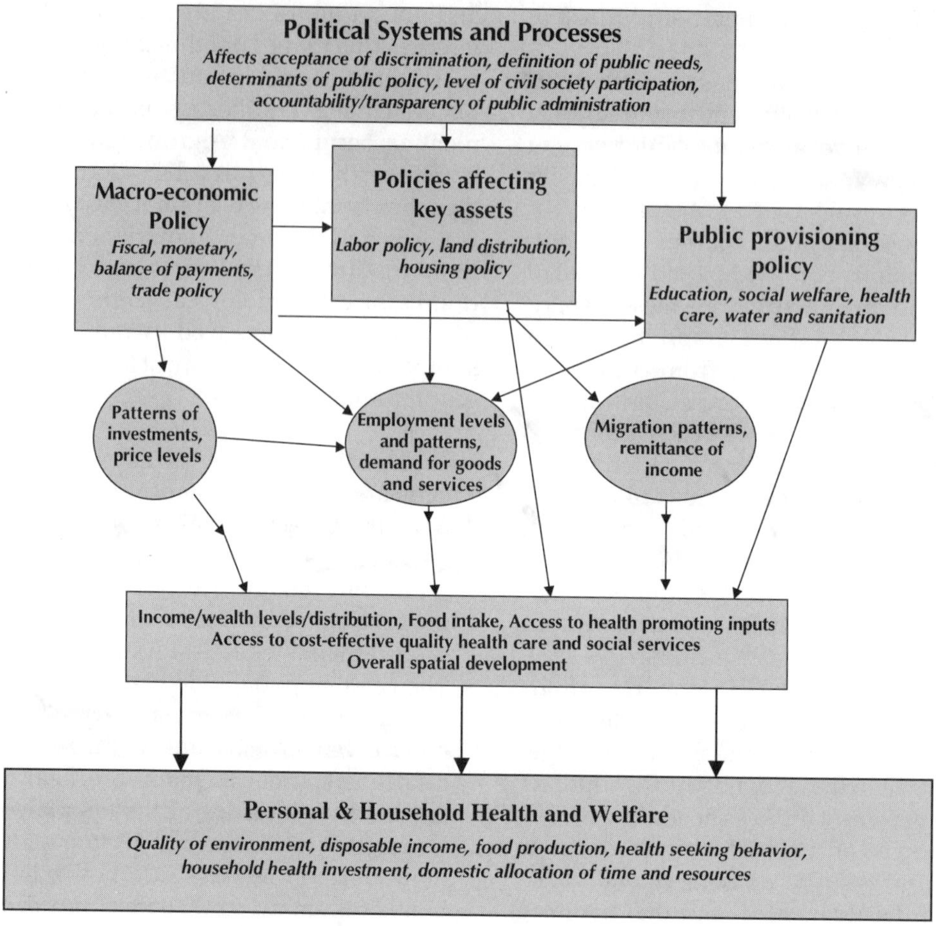

Source: Rockefeller Foundation, Global Health Equity Initiative Report. New York.

care, and utilization of health care services. In Figure 19, a conceptual framework for the identification and analysis of the interrelations between the macro-determinants of health equity is presented. These include the political system and processes (governance as well as level of social and political participation), macroeconomic policy, labor, agrarian and housing policies, as well as policies related to public provisioning of social goods, all of which must be considered to assess the effectiveness of potential interventions to improve health and welfare levels of the population

subgroups presenting avoidable and unfair health disparities.[61]

Many of the democratic governments that are now the norm in LAC are confronting difficulties in satisfying accumulated and unmet demands among their citizens, a situation that in time could compromise governance and stability in the region. Political crises as well as the external economic uncertainty that characterizes the global economy may worsen lev-

[61] Rockefeller Foundation. Global Health Equity Initiative Report. New York, NY: Rockefeller Foundation. In press.

els of social exclusion in Latin America and the Caribbean. There is strong evidence that a major portion of health problems in LAC will not be resolved without transforming our societies into more equitable ones in terms of opportunities for human development of the majority of the population. The prevailing model of economic growth without distribution has led to the growing recognition that the agenda of economic reform of the 1990s must be complemented by a comprehensive package of social and human development initiatives, so that growing health disparities in Latin America and the Caribbean can be successfully addressed.

Based on the conclusions of a recent inter-agency and interregional consultation for the development of future directions in research and policy analysis on health equity,[62] as well as the contributions of Gilson[63] and others, and especially the work that PAHO has been carrying out in the region, the following strategic areas are worthy of consideration as the basis for an agenda to achieve greater equity and fairness in the health of the people of the Americas. These points would also serve as the main areas for the development of technical cooperation activities in health geared towards supporting regional and country level initiatives.

1. *Measurement:* not only to continue the development of instruments and methods for measuring inter-group differences, but also to develop tools to help program managers set targets for reaching the poor and disadvantaged and measure progress towards those targets.
2. *Modification of health services*: it is not sufficient to increase access to existing services; we must also modify services to make them more relevant for the health problems of the poor and marginalized.

3. *Broader determinants of health change*: it is necessary to expand current concern with equity in health care access to other social determinants of health, such as maternal education, water, sanitation, food security, housing and employment, in order to identify effective approaches to improving health.
4. *Advocacy for health equity:* the application of sophisticated statistical techniques for the measurement of intra-country health disparities by socioeconomic class will not have much impact if effective means are not found to introduce this information into the political process to produce programs and policies more relevant for the health of the poor. This includes widening the scope of interaction to include civil society organizations that will assume equity monitoring and "health-watch" roles to influence public policies.
5. *Identification of effective approaches:* Many local policy makers concerned with health equity have already developed effective approaches that need to be recognized and disseminated by international cooperation agencies, a need that would be filled by a systematic search for natural experiments worthy of assessment and suitable for sharing and replicating.

Some of the main conclusions and consequent questions that PAHO's future work may have to address in order to fully develop an effective equity focus for its technical cooperation are highlighted below.

Health care plays a limited role in achieving health status gains and redressing health disparities.

- What are the health systems' "manageable interests" in reducing health disparities?
- Which health interventions have the highest impact on reducing disparities, and for which groups?
- How can "cost-effectiveness" as a criterion for selecting health interventions be complemented by "health equity-inducing potential"? (For example, the provision of water

---

[62] Rockefeller Foundation, World Bank. Health equity consultation summary: Current activities and future directions in health equity. Crystal City, Virginia; 1999.

[63] Gilson L. In defence and pursuit of equity. *Soc Sci Med* 1998; 47: 1891–1896.

and sanitation is not highly cost-effective as measured by DALYs per dollar, but it has a large impact on reducing disparities in health outcomes by greatly improving health of the poor.)

- What health promotion and preventative services (supply driven) are most beneficial to which group?
- How much should be spent on health care, given available resources in each country?

Broader interventions are required to promote health and reduce health disparities.

- What are the health system's "areas of influence" through which it can better exercise advocacy for equity-inducing policies?
- Which groups benefit or lose most, and from which interventions (categorizing by income, ethnicity, sex, education, occupation, place of residence, national origin)?
- How can the "health equity impact" of public policies and interventions be estimated and assessed as part of the policy analysis process?
- What economic policies best promote health development and equity in health?

The analytical approaches used in policy development should reflect these values and better inform policy making and resource allocation.

- How could social weights be incorporated into DALY's and other measurements of burden of disease to reflect social equity values?
- How can the "equity inducing potential" of specific health and other interventions be measured?
- How can existing sources of data, both within and outside the health sector, be better utilized for determining unfair health disparities?
- How can "multi-level" and "multi-source" methods be developed for combining data from different sources for identifying and monitoring health inequities?
- Should the measurement of health dispari-

ties illustrate aggregate differences or differences across individuals? What are the policy implications of each approach?[64]
- What different measurement tools and indicators for health disparities need to be developed and utilized for local level program monitoring? For advocacy purposes? For resource allocation decisions? For target setting and trend analysis? For health impact assessment and evaluation?

Information dissemination is a key input in the work for equity in health, both for advocacy at the top as well as for empowerment below.

- What simple and direct methods and measures can be developed and utilized for quantifying, reporting, and monitoring trends in health disparities?
- How can equity-related information on access to health, both at the local, as well as at the national and global levels, be increased for civil society groups in general and for poor and marginalized groups in particular?
- How can effective participation by civil society and stakeholders in monitoring and advocating for health equity be stimulated?
- How can health equity become a primary national health objective, with clear measurable health goals, both for health related outcomes as well as for determinants?

Health system research must develop broad-based evaluation strategies that allow for the analysis of the equity impact of public policies, including health sector reform.

- How can we develop more effective methods to assess and monitor the impact of financing methods, including user fees, cost recovery and prepayment schemes, decentralization, internal markets, and other reform measures, on different populations?

---

[64] For an alternative viewpoint on the issue of measurement of health disparities across aggregate groups or individuals, see Murray CJL, Gakidou EE, Frenk J. Health inequalities and social group differences: What should we measure? *Bull WHO* 1999; 77 (7): 537–543.

- How can we better identify the impact of non-physical and non-financial barriers on access to health services, such as quality of care (ineffectual poor quality services), gender, cultural factors, national origin, and others?
- How can we better determine objective need, in contrast to perceived need, in order to assess equity in terms of health service utilization?
- What are the health services that require an active "supply" strategy vs. those that are more likely to be spontaneously demanded? How does this difference affect utilization and health outcomes?

ADDITIONAL BIBLIOGRAPHY

Breilh J, Campaña A, Costales P, Granda E, Páez R, Yépez J. Deterioro de la vida: Un instrumento para análisis de prioridades regionales en lo social y la salud. Quito: Corporación Editora Nacional; 1990.

Duncan B, Rummel D, Zelmanowicz A, Mengue S, Santos S, Dalmáz A. Social inequality in mortality in São Paulo State, Brazil. *International Journal of Epidemiology* 1995; 24 (2): 359–365.

Laurell AC. Impacto das políticas sociais e econômicas nos perfis epidemiológicos. In Barata et al. *Eqüidade e saúde: contribuições da epidemiologia*. Rio de Janeiro: Abrasco/FioCruz; 1997.

Mardones-Restat F, Díaz M. Una propuesta de clasificación de las comunas del país: según criterios de riesgo biomédico y socioeconómico para medir la vulnerabilidad infantil. Santiago, Chile: UNICEF; 1990.

Paim J, Costa MC. Decline and Unevenness of Infant Mortality in Salvador, Brazil, 1980–1988. *Bulletin of the Pan American Health Organization* 1993; 27 (1): 1–14.

Velásquez L. Mujer maya y salud. Guatemala: 1994.

Weaver J, Sprout R. In M. Rock (ed.) Twenty-five years of economic development revisited. 1993; 21(11).

POVERTY, HUMAN DEVELOPMENT, AND PUBLIC EXPENDITURE: DEVELOPING ACTIONS FOR GOVERNMENT AND CIVIL SOCIETY

Eduardo Doryan[1]

One dictionary defines poverty as "the state of one who lacks a usual or socially acceptable amount of money or material possessions." Two things are reflected in this definition: first, the standard for what is "socially acceptable" could vary from country to country or between regions of the world; second, poverty is linked not only to money but also to material possessions or assets, including land or any means of production. In the *World Development Report* of 1990, the definition was much more linked to absolute poverty, a condition of life characterized by such malnutrition, illiteracy, and disease as to be beneath any reasonable definition of human decency. This definition brought human outcomes into the definition of poverty. We also have the United Nations Development Program (UNDP) definition of human development. And the Human Development Index (HDI), in particular, looks beyond income and has a more comprehensive definition. Finally, Amartya Sen's definition of poverty is more linked to capabilities, where citizens are well prepared to take advantage of economic opportunities.

The World Bank has conducted a global study, interviewing 60,000 people in 60 coun-

tries throughout the world and capturing the voices of the poor, their definitions of poverty, and how they would like their problems to be resolved. Someone from Ghana said that poverty is "like heat, you cannot see it, you can only feel it. So, to know poverty, you have to go through it." For a poor woman in Moldova, "poverty is pain, it feels like a disease. It attacks a person, not only materially, but also morally. It eats away one's dignity and drives one into total despair."

Keeping in mind the academic definitions of poverty, or at least some of them, and having heard some of the voices of the poor, the international community has established very clear international development goals—halving of the number of people living in poverty by the year 2015; universal access to primary school by the same year; elimination of gender disparities by the year 2005; a two-thirds reduction in infant mortality and mortality in children under 5; and so on. If we look at these goals more closely, we find some direction for action: halving poverty by 2015 is conditional on achieving poverty reducing paths; universal attendance to primary schooling is very much dependent on the quality of teaching in primary schools; gender equality is very much linked to political and economical empowerment of women; and infant mortality in cer-

---

[1] Vice President, World Bank Human Development Network.

tain parts of the world, and probably in certain areas all over the world, is very much conditional on issues such as tackling the spread of HIV/AIDS.

Some of these goals are unlikely to be attained because growth is very volatile, as demonstrated in the Asian crisis and in some of the recent economic crises in Latin America. We also have seen it during natural phenomena such as Hurricane Mitch in Central America. Inequality can rise rapidly in unstable economies, as has occurred in many of the Latin American countries. The adoption and the effective implementation of pro-poor policies and interventions are central, but sometimes are subsumed with the overall macroeconomic policies. Economic policies are a two way street for poverty, however.

There is nothing more effective against poverty than good policies. In Latin America, general economic growth has not led to a decrease in income disparities, and the Gini coefficient for Latin America is much higher than for most other regions of the world. The poor are falling behind in terms of distribution of income; the proportion of income captured by the wealthy grows; and current poverty rates are very much the same as 20 years ago. These results are a reminder of the centrality of human development for all countries.

Although we still have a long way to go, we have learned a great deal about human development and growth. Girls' education is a key factor in health. A study that relates to mothers' education shows that a lack of secondary or higher education has a huge impact on mortality in children under 5 years old (see Table 1). This study also shows that mothers' education is much more important than fathers' in decreasing child mortality. This study points to several important approaches: analyzing policy outcomes, looking beyond health, and finding the linkages and how to make the best investments. Our investments must be directed by an understanding of the dynamics of poverty and human development. This means learning about outcomes for the poorest groups, not just national averages.

A former President of Costa Rica used to tell the following story. "You can have a person lying down with his head in an oven and his legs in a freezer, and the temperature in the belly button is going to be 98.6 degrees. That person is supposed to be in very good health, but probably, that person is very uncomfortable." So, averages are not that useful. We have to think more clearly about the actual meaning of poverty and look at the different income levels in each society.

It is useful, for example to look at the link between education and growth. The average number of years of education for 25-year-olds, grouped by income levels, in Latin America can be divided into ten segments of the population (see Table 2). In Chile, the top decile has twice the years of education as does the lowest decile. In Venezuela the gap between highest and lowest is 2.5 times. The same pattern occurs in countries in different parts of the world. Looking beyond national averages is much needed in development policy.

So, where do we assign more spending? Where we put the resources that are usually meager? Well, that's not an easy question. Health spending alone cannot explain all the variations in health among countries. Nor can income, education, or even disposable income and schooling together. Figure 1 illustrates these discrepancies: the vertical axis shows the deviation from predicted life expectancy in a country; the first upper half of the figure shows deviations from the value predicted on the basis of the country's income and average schooling. France, Singapore, Costa Rica, Honduras, and Sri Lanka, all in the top half of the figures, achieve five years or more of life beyond what would be expected. But Egypt, Ghana, Uganda, the United States, and Zambia, all in the bottom half of the figure, have a life expectancy of about five years lower than expected, given their levels of income and education. The horizontal axis of the figure shows the deviation from predicted percentage of GDP spent in health. Although one might expect that at any level of income and education, higher health spending would

quantitative

TABLE 1. Mortality in children under 5 years old, according to the mother's education.

| Region/country | Mother's educational status | | No education as a multiple of secondary/higher education (col.2/col.3) |
	No education	Secondary/higher education	
Asia/Near East/North Africa			
Indonesia	111	51	2.2
Morocco	91	22	4.1
Pakistan	128	65	2.0
Philippines	152	42	3.6
Turkey	109	30	3.6
Latin America/Caribbean			
Colombia	(74)	25	3.0
Dominican Republic	91	31	2.9
Peru	150	45	3.3
Sub-Saharan Africa			
Burkina Faso	212	87	2.4
Cameroon	198	80	2.5
Ghana	166	69	1.7
Kenya	100	54	1.9
Madagascar	223	114	2.0
Malawi	255	127	2.0
Namibia	97	76	1.3
Niger	334	106	3.2
Nigeria	211	113	1.9
Rwanda	177	94	1.9
Senegal	171	52	3.3
Zambia	204	135	1.5
Unweighted average	164	71	2.3

importance of education

yield better health, all else being equal, there is no evidence of such a relationship. Countries are scattered in all quadrants of the figure, which is partly due to the importance of institutions and policies.

There is much to be done in relation to policies. Probably the best image is that we need developmental cocktails, that is, putting different policy elements together in a way that has a leapfrogging effect, which allows countries to pass through stages of development much more quickly than would be expected from isolated policies.

The *World Development Report* for the upcoming year gives us some premises for policy-making. First, poverty reducing strategies must recognize that appropriately designed combinations of policies will interact in a way that will produce an effect greater than the sum of the individual parts. If we have a robust process of linking different policies, we can actually achieve leapfrogging effects in development. Without such synergistic effects, the 21st century is going to be very difficult for most of the population of Latin America. Another premise for policy-making

TABLE 2. Average years of education for 25-year-olds, by income level, selected countries in Latin America.

Decile	1	2	3	4	5	6	7	8	9	10
Chile	6.24	6.88	7.09	7.40	7.69	8.16	8.47	9.80	10.88	12.83
Brazil	1.98	2.49	2.97	3.41	3.66	4.40	4.49	5.98	7.43	10.53
Mexico	2.14	2.95	3.78	4.15	4.78	5.66	6.06	7.24	8.89	12.13
Peru	3.87	4.17	4.85	5.69	6.60	7.05	7.66	8.28	9.04	10.80
Venezuela	4.66	4.94	5.27	5.72	6.23	6.68	7.20	7.78	8.58	10.81

Quantitative

FIGURE 1. Deviation from predicted life expectancy and deviation from predicted percentage of GDP spent on health, selected countries.

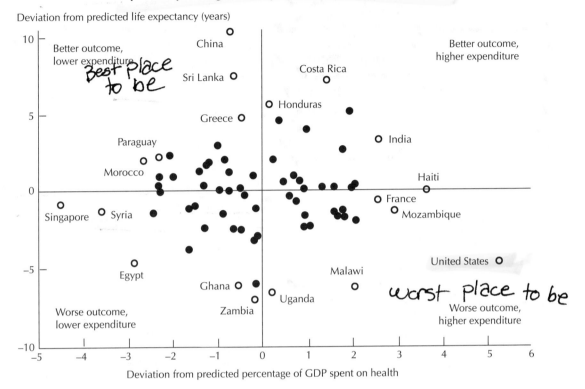

Deviation from predicted percentage of GDP spent on health

is that both growth and inequality are outcomes of economic policy as well as institutional capability, and are subject to external shocks and trends. It is odd that, in the past, analyses have typically looked for mechanical links when investigating growth and inequality jointly, largely ignoring the role of policies. When the role of policies has been investigated, studies have usually looked at growth and inequality separately, yet, the key piece of information, from the point of view of policy makers, is how policies influence both growth and inequality.

The third premise for policy-making is that policies to help the poor should address increasing growth and improving equality at the same time, or at least mitigating inequality by generating growth with pro-poor measures. Policy makers should take into account (1) the

effects that different health care system financing methods have on improving health status, (2) how to ensure equity, (3) the linking of microeconomic and macroeconomic efficiency, (4) the enhancement of clinical effectiveness, (5) the improvement of care quality and consumer satisfaction, and (6) the assessment of the system's long-run financial stability, as they have important consequences for equity across income groups. They must consider the amount of revenue that can be raised, and losses in consumer welfare and production generated by different revenue raising techniques. These considerations are at the core of how to tackle the problems of poverty, inequity, and development in our countries.

The political economy of health policies and human development policies are going to be very important. In the first place, there is a need to spend more, but with the caveat that spending is not enough if developmental cocktails and leapfrogging effects are not present in policy prescriptions. Second, health service outputs are needed. Finally, we need to move from outputs to outcomes. This third category relates to the effects that health expenditures have on health outcomes, and is tied to intersectoral factors such as education, water and sanitation, and women's status, because health services are just one factor among many that determines the population health status.

This presents difficulties from a political point of view, because the international financial community, which lends money, as well as many organizations, have very sectoral approaches. Those who work in health deal with the Minister of Health, others deal with the Minister of Education, and others deal with the Minister of Labor. Pulling together intersectoral development packages is not easy, and without an articulated approach, it will be impossible to prepare those cocktails and achieve the leapfrogging effects as we would like.

The "Voices of the Poor" study showed that there was a comprehensive view of development. From villagers in a republic in Central Asia we heard, "our problems are lack of jobs and money; high price of food, clothes, and health care; and lack of shops. Besides, we don't have training manuals, there is no high school, no public baths, and most important, there is no drinking water. We have to buy it and then keep it for a long time, so it goes bad, but we still use it."

Development is moving from ill being to well being. The 60,000 people who were interviewed repeated that they have a sense of powerlessness, weak social relations, material lack and poverty, physical weakness, and insecurity—ill being. And what they wanted was good social relations, security, physical well being, enough for a good life, and freedom of choice and action. Well being embodies much more than how to overcome poverty; it is related to equity, but it is also holistic in relation to the experience of life.

Next year's *World Development Report* will focus on three core issues. Empowerment is the first, and includes addressing economic, social, political, and institutional inequalities that prevent the poor and disadvantaged from having access to and influence over policies and interventions that influence their lives. The second important issue is security, livelihood, and risk management policies, including those related to natural disasters and economic shock, which poor nations will increasingly face in the global economy and which has always trapped the poor in poor countries in poverty. The third major component is opportunity and putting in place the conditions for investment and sustainable economic development. The poor must participate fully in the creation of such policies, and the policies must not degrade the environment or increase risk and vulnerability. These issues are not hierarchical, but rather are interrelated components of our overall framework for poverty reduction and equity. This framework clearly cuts across the more conventional sectoral framework of interventions. For example, health affects all three dimensions, even as each of the three dimensions affect each other.

From a policy-making perspective, we have seen that empowerment, opportunity, and risk management are core elements of equitable development. Whenever countries have used the benefits of growth to finance basic health care and access to education for all, and when countries have put in place incentive structures and complementary investments to insure that better health and education lead to higher incomes, the poor have doubly benefited. They are healthier and better educated, and they have increased their consumption. We must not only finance basic education and access to health, but also have a system in place that feeds back those investments into more productivity and growth. Such an approach will create a virtuous circle and not reproduce a vicious circle in which financing is not increased nor linked to the economic nor productive strategies. Those cycles of growth are followed by economic shocks that create a vicious circle that degrades health and education indicators. A final corollary is that moving from income, which has been the traditional focus of equity, to multi-dimensional views of poverty has policy consequences. Even if incomes do not increase, policies that improve the health of individuals and increase their capacity to absorb and exchange information improve the quality of their lives. Health must be put in the context of poverty reduction and linked to education, social protection, and other aspects of human development. The effect of health must also be considered in the context of its influence on empowerment, opportunity, and risk management, and we must find ways to pull together such policies and finance them in a way that really tackles the key aspects that affect and improve the quality of life and the well being of the poor.

POVERTY, EQUITY, AND HEALTH: SOME RESEARCH FINDINGS

Adam Wagstaff[1] is an economist

more qualitative

This chapter will deal with research that is of general interest both to the industrialized and countries that are not part of the Organization for Economic Cooperation and Development (OECD). It will cover poverty, equity, and health, and how we can link research to policy-making. Let's start with the goals we are trying to pursue in the health sector and how these relate to the notions of poverty and equity. I have listed here two broad goals, goals that keep coming up time and time again in health documents.

The first is, obviously, the improvement of health; not just improving health, however, but also improving it equitably. Now that means different things to different people. It would mean, for example, at least, making sure that you promote the health of the poor and, possibly, even more strongly making sure that the health of the poor improves faster than the health of the non-poor. This would probably entail two things: promoting access to health care, especially among the worse-off, and focusing on the nonmedical determinants of health—those things that lie outside of what we traditionally think of as the health care sector.

A second strand of policy objectives in the health field involves income protection; essentially, making sure the poor don't suffer large

reductions in their living standards through out-of-pocket payments and through loss of earnings when they fall sick. The second element of this income protection goal is to build risk-pooling mechanisms that result in protection payments being linked to ability to pay. As we'll see in a moment, there are different ways of providing people with protection against out-of-pocket payments, and each has different distributional consequences.

Let me start with the income protection goal. A poignant example of the need for income protection is described in "Voices of the Poor," in which a 26-year-old man from Vietnam moved from being the richest member of his community to being the poorest member of his community, simply because he incurred very large health care expenses associated with his daughter's illness. If you read "Voices of the Poor," this is an issue that comes through very strongly. When people think about designing health care systems, the poor feel very strongly that one of the important dimensions of that debate is how to protect their income and livelihood.

Among OECD countries, with the exception of Portugal, very few countries raise more than 20% of their revenues from out-of-pocket payments. Among non-OECD countries, the picture is quite different. In Bangladesh, for example, more than 60% of health care revenues are paid from out-of-pocket.

One issue, then, is how regressive these payments are. What 'regressiveness' means is

---

[1] Professor of Economics, University of Sussex, U.K. and Principal Economist, World Bank's Development Economics Research Group and Human Development Network

Regressive → everyone taxed equally
Progressive → poor pay less than rich
more towards this ↙ pay smaller percentages
better

what proportion of a family's income these payments represent. If, as we move up through the income distribution, the proportion of income spent on out-of-pocket payments declines, then you have a regressive structure. If, on the other hand, it increases—that is, the rich pay a larger share of their income in out-of-pocket payments than the poor—that is a progressive structure. Most of the evidence on this issue comes from OECD countries, but we now are getting some numbers in from the non-OECD countries. What is emerging is that there are two distinct groups of countries. There are countries such as China, Rumania, and Bulgaria, where people are seeking care and obtaining care, but paying for it in a very severe way. For example, there is a very high degree of regressiveness in the out-of-pocket payment structure in China. At the other end of the spectrum, we have countries where out-of-pocket payments are actually slightly progressive, as they absorb a larger share of the income of wealthy households than they do of poor household incomes. There are two possibilities here, of course. One is that people who cannot afford care are simply not getting it; the other possibility is that they are getting it, but there are systems or mechanisms in place to reduce the impact of out-of-pocket payments.

Regressiveness is only one part of the story. Another part of the story is whether households are plunged into poverty through out-of-pocket payments. According to our estimates, many households fall into poverty through out-of-pocket payments, and the tendency for this is greater among those who don't have insurance. So, it is not just a question of regresiveness; it is a question of households being put into poverty through out-of-pocket payments.

How can we provide households with protection against out-of-pocket payments? Different countries raise their health care revenues in different ways. We have some countries, specifically the United States and Switzerland, which have a very strong emphasis on private insurance, while the Netherlands has some emphasis on private insurance. Social insurance, which is, of course, very common in Latin America, represents a big portion of expenditures in Latin American countries, but also in countries like France, Germany, and the Netherlands. The rest of the expenditures are generated through tax revenues.

These different ways of providing households with protection have different distributional consequences in relation to the income that households have to spend on things other than health care and also on private health care. If we're interested both in the consumption possibilities for private health care as well as the extent to which households can purchase things other than health care—if we're concerned, for example, about poverty—then these distributional consequences are important to take into account.

In the United Kingdom, direct taxes contribute progressively towards the total financing burden. As a matter of fact, this also is the case in Ireland, Egypt, and Bulgaria. If we also consider indirect taxes—as we know from our studies of OECD countries—countries such as the UK and Spain, which greatly emphasize indirect taxes, these structures become regressive, which tends to reduce or offset the progressivity of direct taxes. Interestingly, what emerges for some of the non-OECD countries is that indirect taxes actually end up being progressive. This is not true in Mexico, where the scheme is marginally regressive, but it is true of those other countries. What is occurring there is that those countries are relying on a graded structure where luxury items are taxed at a higher rate. In the case of social insurance, the level of progressivity and regressivity pretty much depends on what the scheme is. In the Netherlands, Germany, and Mexico, for example, social insurance programs are regressive. In countries like China, they are actually progressive.

If we substitute private insurance as the financing mechanism, we see that in the two big countries where this is an important source of finance, the system is very regressive. In other countries it is regressive, too, but either because it is less important, or because it is not as regressive, it doesn't feature so prominently in this chart. In almost all the OECD countries, out-of-pocket payments are regressive, and in the non-OECD countries it varies a little bit. In countries like Egypt, out-of-pocket payments are progressive, but in countries like China, where they're very important, they are very regressive.

EQUITABLE HEALTH PROMOTION

Poorer people are more often sick, sick for longer periods of time than the less poor, so, they just sleep and groan.

—Malawan woman, quoted in
"Voices of the Poor"

Is the burden of illness unequally distributed in these countries? In almost all these countries inequalities and mortality in children under 5 years old are concentrated among the poor to a statistically significant degree. There are differences across countries: the degree to which mortality in children under 5 is concentrated among the poor is not fixed; it varies across countries. Brazil, for example, comes out with an especially high degree of inequality.

In the case of stunting, countries like Peru, Brazil, and Nicaragua, which we know have very unequal income distributions, also have a very unequal distribution of childhood stunting. The poor in these countries are much, much more likely to be stunted than the non-poor. What can we do to remove these inequalities, or at least promote the health of the poor?

Another quote from "Voices of the Poor" points out the importance of access to health care. "It is precisely those who are most exposed to health risks, whose work entails the greatest risks of accidents or debilitation, and who are most dependent on the strength of their bodies—in short, those who need health care most—who are the least able to afford and obtain it."

Is health care distributed unequally? In most of the OECD countries, it is actually the poor who get more health care than the non-poor. One might claim, in response, that this is not taking into account the fact that the poor need more health care. If we standardize the distributions, the pro-poorness is reduced substantially, but not eliminated, except in the United States and Switzerland. In other words, we don't have to throw up our hands in despair and say it's never going to be possible to get health care to the poor. There are countries in the world that manage to do it.

In China, the picture is quite different from the picture for the OECD countries. Inpatient care in particular is highly skewed, not towards the poor, but towards the better-off. It is a less pronounced disparity in the case of outpatient visits, but overall what we see is a picture where the Chinese are failing to get health care to the poor.

One might say, well, that's sometimes because the rich choose to purchase more, but let's look at what happens to the public subsidy, which surely ought to be going to the poor. There are some data from a variety of different countries that show how the poor compare to the non-poor, showing the concentration index for public subsidies. There are many countries where the subsidies are actually going to the better-off, including Brazil and Peru. Some Latin American countries seem, on this criterion, to be doing quite well, but what I suspect we're picking up right here are only the ministry of health's subsidy, not the subsidies going through the social security systems. Data from Peru and from Honduras are much more comprehensive, and I think you'd get a much better picture from those data.

Why do the poor get less, then? Well, if we look at econometric work, and this is backed up by consultation studies with the poor, what's going on seems to be lack of income, low education, poor understanding of what there is to be gained from the system, money prices, and insurance status, all of which are clearly important. But things we tend to forget include distance to travel, ease of transportation, waiting time, and opening hours. Very often the poor will say, "I don't go to the clinic, because when I get there it's never open." Quality of care is fundamentally important and comes through very strongly in some recent econometric work. Often the poor don't go to clinics because when they get there, even if the place is open, the clinic has no drugs. They prefer to pay out-of-pocket and go somewhere that is closer and well stocked. Staff attitudes also are important. The poor complain about things like being slapped by staff or, if not being physically abused, of being verbally abused.

The fundamental point, though, is that health care is never going to be enough. Another person cited in "Voices of the Poor" says, "the poor frequently are disadvantaged by where they live due to geographical isolation; marginal land; . . . lack of transport, sanitation, water, and other services; isolation from information; environmental hazards; inadequate shelter; insecure rights to land; physical insecurity and crime. . . ." These are all important for health itself, not just in their own right.

Some figures from Cebu, the Philippines, show us the degree to which different determinants of health are concentrated among the poor or the non-poor. It's much more likely, for example, that poor households are those that will have no water supply. Mothers who only have elementary education are much more likely to be among the poor; households that don't have a toilet are much more likely to be amongst the poor; the poor take longer to travel to a health center; and poor women are more likely to have more pregnancies. In the case of Cebu, it seems that the local facilities in poor areas are actually more likely to offer immunization than those in the non-poor areas. Corn and rice seem to have slightly higher prices in poor areas. Among richer households, there tends to be access to a greater number of nurses in local facilities, mothers are more likely to have a high school education, and the better-off are more likely to have some form of health insurance.

We can estimate the impact of these factors on childhood survival using a survival model. Being a boy in Cebu is not that good in terms of childhood survival prospects, nor is having an old mother when you're born or having a mother who has had a lot of children by the time you are born. If you have a mother who's well educated, that's good for survival. Living in a low-income household is bad for survival, and not having a toilet is bad for survival. Having health insurance is good, and having a local facility that offers an immunization program also is good for your survival chances.

Now, none of these things come through as particularly surprising. You'd say, "but I knew all that, anyway, and I also knew that the poor didn't have toilets and that they had to travel further, and so on." But what we can do with these two sets of numbers is put them together and try and get a handle on this question of how important health care is. We say health care is just one of the factors, and we feel we ought to say that, but how important is it—50%, 60%? More precisely, if we were to reduce the inequalities that we saw a moment ago in each of these various determinants of health, what impact could we have on inequalities in health outcomes?

We saw, for example, that the poor tend to have to travel further, and it takes them longer to reach a health facility. What would happen if we had the poor and all the bottom four quintiles traveling the same amount of time as the top quintile? Not a lot. This shows that we get a slight reduction in the overall average rate and a slight improvement in the inequality, but it's not exactly something to write home about.

What if we improve the quality of medical facilities? In this case, because it's actually the poor areas that have better immunization facilities, the exercise brings everybody else down to the level of the top quintile. Not surprisingly, we actually worsen the outcome.

What if we could give everybody the same insurance coverage as the top quintile has? We actually get a little bit further in the right direction. But if we could give the poor and the bottom four quintiles generally the same sanitation conditions as the rich top quintile, we would actually achieve quite a big jump.

If we could equalize mothers' schooling, and stop poor women from having children late in life and from having so many of them, we also would achieve a big impact.

The final exercise is to look at the effect of equalizing income distribution. Holding everything else constant, we would achieve a very large reduction in the average rates and a very big reduction in the inequalities. This gives us a sense of humility, if you like, by demonstrating how and how much we need to cooperate with people in other sectors, because it's not just simply that there are other things that matter. It's more important than that; it's that these other things matter tremendously when we are thinking about improving outcomes of the poor.

We've learned quite a lot about income protection: out-of-pocket payments very often hit the poor hardest and very often cause poverty. We can have different ways of linking protection to ability to pay and they have different income distribution consequences. We need to think those through. In the area of improving the health of the population we see dramatic differences between poor and nonpoor. We see a difference between the OECD countries and the non-OECD countries in terms of who gets health care and who gets the subsidies to the health system. And when it comes to looking at the nonmedical determinants of health, the results we saw for Cebu suggest we need to think very carefully about the relative importance of different types of inequality for reducing health inequality. Increasing access to health services, promoting health insurance coverage, and so on, are definitely important, but there are other big things we need to really worry about, too.

2 biggest things to improve → education & sanitation

Equidad, Minorías Étnicas y Derechos Humanos Fundamentales

Pilar Córdova[1]

Mientras escuchaba las presentaciones anteriores sentía una gran preocupación, porque yo no soy una técnica experta en salud. Podría decirse que soy una aficionada, una persona que lucha por la construcción de equidad para los hombres y mujeres de mi país y de la Región. ¿Por qué estoy aquí entonces? Hace unos tres años vine al Banco Interamericano de Desarrollo con el afán de contribuir a la discusión acerca de la problemática de las minorías étnicas no solo de Colombia, sino de América Latina en general. Logré interesar al Doctor Iglesias, Presidente del Banco Interamericano Desarrollo, sobre la necesidad de asignar recursos y realizar estudios diferenciales de estas poblaciones en la Región, no solo de los grupos indígenas sino también de los afro-colombianos. En esa ocasión, visité la OPS y conocí a Cristina Torres, a quien también le planteé el tema —que me parece muy importante desde la perspectiva de la salud— de las diferencias que deberían existir en relación con las minorías, en este caso negras o afro-colombianas, o afro-americanas, dado que en la Región ya existía un interés o una intención diferente con respecto a las comunidades indígenas. Hoy estoy aquí para compartir con ustedes una serie de inquietudes, proponer alternativas y, sobre todo, aportar elementos para la discusión y la preparación de agendas públicas.

Creo que al hablar de factores de inequidad se hace referencia al tema de los derechos humanos, de los derechos fundamentales que no solo se asocian a los derechos civiles y políticos, sino a los que han sido denominados derechos de segunda generación o derechos blandos, es decir, los derechos sociales, económicos y culturales. Esto me lleva al tema de la justicia social moderna, una de las cuestiones importantes de este fin de siglo, y a indagar sobre la forma más efectiva de eliminar las inequidades y construir sistemas de salud igualitarios, universales, accesibles, eficaces y eficientes. El concepto actual de justicia social se basa en dos elementos fundamentales: en primer lugar, la distribución o desconcentración de la riqueza, y en segundo término, una cuestión novedosa e interesante: el reconocimiento de la diferencia y de la participación. Juntos, estos elementos constituyen un sistema integral.

Esta idea de la justicia social nos conduce a la conceptualización del estado social y democrático de derecho. Así, a finales del siglo XX, al concepto de estado liberal y utilitarista se le contrapone el de estado social y democrático de derecho, con sus tres elementos fundamentales: el objetivo social, la concepción democrática del poder, y la sujeción a la ley. Esta es la concepción moderna del estado social de derecho, y ella nos lleva necesariamente al tema de los derechos humanos, de los derechos fundamentales que forman parte esen-

---

[1] Senadora, Colombia.

cial del nuevo estado social, democrático y de derecho.

Estos derechos fundamentales humanos, sociales, económicos y culturales surgen como respuesta a las inequidades que imperaron en el siglo pasado y que todavía están presentes en este siglo: la pobreza, la exclusión, la marginalidad, la falta de participación y, sobre todo, la violencia. Hace unos dos o tres años, en Costa Rica, participé en la presentación del informe sobre el desarrollo humano. En esa ocasión expresé la necesidad de incorporar el fenómeno de la violencia, porque, a mi juicio, no se puede hablar en términos generales de desarrollo humano sin incluir una problemática que está desgarrando a muchos de nuestros países. No tener en cuenta la violencia impide medir en forma apropiada el índice de desarrollo humano. La propuesta no recibió buena acogida en ese momento; sin embargo, vemos que el último informe de desarrollo humano ha incorporado el elemento de la violencia, que es un factor de inequidad, como una de las mediciones reales del índice de desarrollo humano.

Los factores de inequidad que acabo de mencionar no representan más que la incapacidad de lograr la igualdad. Cuando hablamos de lograr la equidad, no tenemos que ir muy lejos, porque la pobreza, la exclusión, la violencia, la marginalidad y la discriminación son los fenómenos subyacentes de las causas estructurales que generan inequidad. Estas causas tienen mucho que ver con la mala distribución del ingreso y la imposibilidad de participación, y todo ello se relaciona con la construcción del poder político y con lo que alguien ha denominado el buen gobierno. Los factores de inequidad mencionados se vinculan estrechamente con la corrupción, fenómeno que no puede considerarse de manera superficial porque expresa las falencias de una sociedad que elimina la disponibilidad de recursos que posibilitarían la construcción de equidad e igualdad.

Creo que una de las metas del fin de siglo y una de las discusiones importantes del próximo milenio es el reconocimiento de esos derechos sociales, económicos y culturales como derechos fundamentales. No es lo mismo hablar de estos derechos fundamentales como derechos humanos, pues son diferentes en la medida en que los estados no les conceden a los derechos fundamentales —el derecho a la participación política, al reconocimiento de los derechos civiles, el derecho de reunión, de opinión— igual importancia que a los derechos sociales, económicos y culturales que se relacionan precisamente con la salud, la educación, la vivienda y el derecho a la diferencia cultural y a la recreación.

Por eso decía —y me parece importante hacer esta digresión aquí— que los estados tienen la obligación de observar esos derechos fundamentales, no únicamente la obligación de acatarlos, sino de no omitirlos, incluso bajo sanciones no solo nacionales sino internacionales. Los países deben establecer progresivamente los derechos sociales, económicos y culturales, y deben arbitrar los recursos necesarios para que la población cuente con sistemas de salud universales, eficientes y eficaces. Si bien es importante hablar de los factores sociales de inequidad, es necesario ubicarlos en el contexto de una concepción filosófica del estado social democrático de derecho, que tiene un objetivo social, está sujeto a la ley y, además, posee una concepción democrática del poder. Todo ello en el marco de los derechos sociales, económicos y culturales que han sido los elementos contrapuestos para eliminar los factores de inequidad que aún se observan en la sociedad de fin de siglo.

Es importante hacer estas observaciones iniciales, porque los derechos sociales, económicos y culturales se materializan en sistemas de salud, de educación, de vivienda, de recreación, y estos sistemas deben estar respaldados jurídicamente por un marco constitucional, por leyes y disposiciones legales, y por planes y programas de desarrollo. Los sistemas y el marco constitucional y legal poseen un objetivo último que es el ser humano, es decir, deben posibilitar condiciones de vida dignas, igualdad de oportunidades y reconocimiento —del que forman parte la diferencia y la participación— y, sobre todo, el acceso sostenido a los sistemas de salud, educación, vivienda y recreación.

En relación con los derechos sociales, económicos y culturales y, en este caso específico, con el tema de la salud, debe hacerse una consideración muy de fondo. Cuando se habla de la universalidad de los derechos, se hace referencia a la generalidad de los derechos sin hacer abstracciones de tipo regional, local, étnico o de género. Hay que recalcar que la idea de universalidad no supone dejar de reconocer lo étnico, lo cultural, lo genérico, lo regional o lo local. Sin desconocer la importancia de la universalidad y de la igualdad de oportunidades, creo que no reconocer esos factores implica quitar visibilidad a grandes sectores poblacionales, o a la mitad de la población que somos las mujeres, generando inequidades en la pobreza, en la exclusión, en la violencia o en la marginalidad.

En Colombia, desde hace seis o siete años, algunos sectores —mujeres o minorías étnicas, como en mi caso— comenzamos a reflexionar sobre la necesidad de que se materialice una discusión muy importante sobre el derecho a la diferencia por parte de grupos como los afro-colombianos y las poblaciones indígenas del país. Esto coincide con la discusión sobre la Constituyente, que dio como resultado la formulación de una nueva Constitución en la que se dice que Colombia "es un país multi-étnico y pluricultural". Se trata de una discusión interesante en la medida en que comprende no solo las obligaciones del Estado hacia estos grupos, que no habían sido hasta ahora reconocidos en la Constitución, sino también los derechos adquiridos por ellos frente a las exigencias del estado. Esto supuso discusiones arduas e interesantes y, al mismo tiempo, avances significativos, ya que condujeron a la aprobación de artículos específicos sobre la población afro-colombiana y la población indígena desde el punto de vista étnico.

En cuanto a la elaboración de planes de desarrollo, tanto en lo que respecta al país en general como a las poblaciones afro-colombianas en particular, la problemática ha sido enriquecida de manera importante. No sé qué grado de conocimiento tengan muchos de ustedes acerca de esta discusión de lo étnico, que va mucho más allá de la polémica de los años sesenta y setenta sobre los derechos civiles y políticos de los grupos afro-americanos en los Estados Unidos. En Colombia y en otras regiones de América Latina ya no se trata solamente del reconocimiento de poder elegir y ser elegido, sino del derecho a un desarrollo diferenciado. Todo esto ha conducido a la sanción de la Ley 70, o Ley de Negritudes, y a la puesta en marcha de un programa de cooperación internacional llamado Plan Pacífico-BID, que posibilitó la asignación de recursos muy importantes en materia de salud en las zonas de la Región donde los grupos afro-colombianos tienen ascendencia y presencia. No obstante, aun cuando los resultados no fueron los esperados, porque esto sucedió en la época del cólera, lo importante de la experiencia es que desde una perspectiva de política pública, con una visión de nación y a partir de la discusión sobre la plurietnia o la multi-culturalidad, se elaboró un plan cabal de desarrollo que fue sometido a la cooperación internacional y discutido con las comunidades, y se pudieron arbitrar los recursos.

En efecto, en esos momentos una epidemia gravísima de cólera azotaba toda una región de población negra que antes no había tenido visibilidad para las políticas públicas, y desde la perspectiva del gobierno, del Ejecutivo e incluso el Legislativo, tampoco existían las condiciones necesarias para arbitrar este tipo de recursos. Hoy, por ejemplo, de esa Ley 70 de Negritudes se han desprendido otras disposiciones. Así, en el Plan Nacional de Desarrollo se establece la obligación de que las comunidades afro-colombianas también analicen y aprueben un Plan de Desarrollo precisamente para esta población. El Plan de Desarrollo Nacional no se puede aprobar si antes el Plan de Desarrollo de las Comunidades Afro-colombianas no ha sido discutido, aprobado e incorporado en el marco del primero. Esto es muy interesante como discusión teórica sobre el estado y la construcción de la nacionalidad, y sobre todo es interesante en el sentido de que este tipo de perspectivas de políticas públicas diferenciadas por regiones, por etnias o por género, puede evitar conflictos en la sociedad, porque en la medida en que estos grupos (o la mitad de la humanidad que somos las mujeres) no sean visibles en las políticas públicas, no se posibilita la convivencia, y, sobre todo, el goce de los derechos sociales, económicos y culturales que eviten esos bolsones de inequidad.

Aun cuando Colombia tiene uno de los marcos legislativos más interesantes de la Región en lo que se refiere a lo étnico (no solo lo indígena), todavía falta mucho por avanzar. Con respecto a la cuestión de la africanidad, en muchos países de América Latina ni siquiera se reconoce la existencia de poblaciones negras, como ocurre en el Uruguay, o en el Paraguay. Incluso en el Brasil, que tiene 80 millones de negros, las políticas públicas son generales y no atienden a las diferencias culturales. Es más, aunque no soy médica, me atrevería a decir que las enfermedades que afectan a una persona mestiza o blanca no son las mismas que las que afectan a una persona negra o indígena. Igualmente, aplicar las políticas de manera general sin "tranversalizarlas", sin focalizarlas (aunque no me gusta este término) y sin diferenciar, termina por quitar visibilidad a las personas, generar más pobreza e impedir el acceso a la salud y a los sistemas de salud, porque sus enfermedades ni siquiera son reconocidas en las políticas públicas como afecciones propias de una etnia, una raza o una condición de la Región.

Para finalizar, considero que no solo es importante hablar de las políticas públicas, los planes de desarrollo o el buen gobierno, es decir, de sistemas eficaces y sin corrupción, sino también discutir algo que mencionó hace muy poco Kofi Annan cuando hablaba de la paz, el desarrollo y la desigualdad horizontal. La desigualdad horizontal se da cuando en un país los mismos recursos se concentran en unas pocas personas o regiones, desconociéndose o ignorando a otras minorías que existen en el país, o desconociendo a más de

la mitad de la población que somos las mujeres. La desigualdad horizontal genera muchos conflictos y más desigualdad, y es un elemento que debe agregarse a los factores sociales de inequidad. Los recursos en el país no se aplican en forma adecuada debido a ese desconocimiento y falta de visibilidad de sectores marginales de la población, o marginados del desarrollo. Por eso es importante hablar sobre el buen gobierno, en el sentido de lo que son los desarrollos legislativos, los marcos constitucionales, el reconocimiento de los derechos sociales, económicos y culturales, la visibilidad pública y política de los pobres, la marginalidad, la exclusión, todos ellos factores subyacentes a la construcción de igualdad.

Es muy importante, y no solo necesario, que esto se conozca, que se coloque en la agenda pública y que se discuta, a fin de asignar mejor los recursos una vez identificadas las necesidades fundamentales. Dos de las cosas más importantes que he escuchado aquí en la mañana de hoy, se refieren a los derechos sociales fundamentales que no se pueden convertir en derechos de mercancías: el derecho a la educación y el derecho a la salud. Creo que hay que avanzar del parroquialismo y de las barreras mentales que tenemos entre países, o las barreras no tanto ideológicas sino territoriales, para decir que es importantísimo que esos recursos se arbitren en forma apropiada. Que el presupuesto, cuando se discuta, tenga la importancia y la implicancia necesaria para saber si es más importante el desarrollo y la paz que la guerra y la dedicación de recursos a otros destinos que no son los fundamentales para los países.

En cuanto a la cooperación internacional, creo que tiene muchas tareas por delante. En primer lugar, la tarea de informar a las regiones, a los países, a las comunidades. En segundo lugar, en el caso de las minorías étnicas, capacitar. Nuestra gente tiene la posibilidad de participar en la discusión del plan de desarrollo, de elaborar su propio plan, pero no sabe cómo hacerlo porque carece de los instrumentos necesarios; en lo que se refiere a la salud, no cuenta con la información pertinente. Las comunidades no poseen los conocimientos que les permiten discutir el plan de desarrollo y demandar la asignación de recursos para que la fiebre amarilla, por ejemplo, se pueda tratar y erradicar, haciendo hincapié en las diferencias étnicas y regionales. En tercer lugar, creo que hay un tema que debe figurar en todas las agendas de cooperación internacional, trátese de mujeres, de minorías étnicas o de países pobres, y es el seguimiento de los recursos y la determinación de su implicancia en relación con los objetivos que se persiguen.

Si se está tratando de acabar con la pobreza, entonces cómo es que esa pobreza se va a acabar con esos recursos de la cooperación. Si se habla de que las minorías étnicas, que son las más pobres, las que viven en las zonas de mayor descuido estatal, las más enfermas, cómo es que esos recursos de salud se están removiendo de esas causas que los vuelve más enfermos y más pobres, es decir, cuáles son los resultados finales que arrojó esa asignación de recursos y si los objetivos realmente se están cumpliendo. Y cuáles son las sanciones que habrán de aplicarse en un momento determinado. Esa es una discusión que quisiera dejar abierta, porque no sé en realidad a quién se sanciona, si a la pobre gente, que es la que no está recibiendo los recursos, o al estado, que no es capaz de utilizarlos para eliminar las causas de inequidad y lograr la construcción de igualdad. Muchísimas gracias.

PART 2

PRIORITIES FOR INCORPORATING EQUITY INTO TECHNICAL COOPERATION IN HEALTH IN THE AMERICAS

La Medición de las Desigualdades en Salud: Algunos Ejemplos de la Región de las Américas

George A. O. Alleyne,[1] Carlos Castillo-Salgado,[2] Cristina Schneider,[2] Oscar J. Mujica,[2] Enrique Loyola[2] y Manuel Vidaurre[2]

INTRODUCCIÓN

Durante el último decenio, varios de los principales indicadores de salud de las Américas han mostrado una considerable mejoría, resultante de factores sociales, culturales y tecnológicos favorables, así como de una mayor disponibilidad y acceso a los servicios y programas de salud. Sin embargo, la mejoría no ha sido igual para todos los países, ni para todos los grupos humanos de un país cualquiera. Diversas publicaciones de la Organización Panamericana de la Salud (OPS) documentan estas desigualdades (1–4).

El logro de la equidad en salud es fundamental en la Región de las Américas, en particular en América Latina y el Caribe, cuya distribución del ingreso es la más inequitativa del mundo (5) (Figura 1). La disminución de las desigualdades y el logro de la meta de salud para todos a mediano plazo constituyen un desafío y un compromiso para los gobiernos, la Organización Mundial de la Salud (OMS), la OPS, y otros organismos e instituciones que actúan en este campo.

La obtención de evidencia objetiva sobre las diferencias en las condiciones de salud y de vida representa el primer paso para distinguir las inequidades en salud (6). Desigualdad e inequidad no son sinónimos: la inequidad es una desigualdad injusta y evitable, y por ello es un concepto crucial para la definición de políticas públicas de salud. El análisis de las inequidades requiere un conocimiento de sus causas determinantes y un juicio acerca de la evitabilidad y la probable injusticia de dichas causas.

Este capítulo tiene el propósito de mostrar algunas evidencias objetivas de las desigualdades en materia de salud entre los países de la Región, y su asociación con indicadores socioeconómicos. También se propone ilustrar el empleo de algunos instrumentos clásicos para la medición de las desigualdades, por medio de la presentación y análisis de algunos ejemplos escogidos.

LAS DESIGUALDADES DE LA SITUACIÓN DE SALUD EN LAS AMÉRICAS

Los instrumentos que se emplean en este artículo para medir las desigualdades en sa-

---

[1] Director, Organización Panamericana de la Salud.
[2] Programa Especial de Análisis de Salud, Organización Panamericana de la Salud.

FIGURA 1. Distribución del ingreso por quintiles, varias regiones del Mundo, 1990.

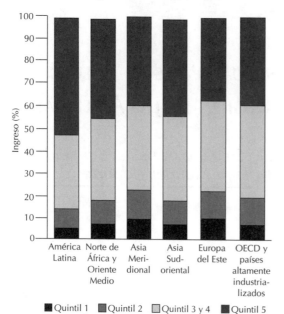

Fuente: Banco Mundial; Sistema de Información Técnica, Programa Especial de Análisis de Salud, Organización Panamericana de la Salud.

lud se basan en datos de morbilidad, mortalidad y factores asociados al estado de salud contenidos en el Sistema de Información Técnica de la OPS. Hay varias revisiones metodológicas importantes en este campo, de las cuales las más conocidas son los trabajos de Mackenbach y Kunst (7, 8), y de Wagstaff, Paci y van Doorslaer (9).

La comparación de la situación de salud entre grupos socioeconómicos puede expresarse tanto en términos absolutos (en unidades de desigualdad) como relativos (en relación con un valor de referencia). Otra opción metodológica consiste en el empleo de medidas para evaluar el efecto de la situación socioeconómica sobre las condiciones de salud, o su impacto. La diferencia esencial entre ambas opciones es que las medidas de impacto toman en cuenta el estado real de la situación socioeconómica y ponderan los cambios que pueden esperarse en la condición de sa-

lud como resultado de posibles intervenciones; por tal motivo, estas medidas son especialmente importantes en relación con la toma de decisiones y el diseño de políticas públicas encaminadas al logro de la equidad.[3]

EFECTO DE LAS DESIGUALDADES

Los indicadores de efecto se utilizan con frecuencia para documentar las inequidades en salud. El informe Black (10), un innovador trabajo de los años ochenta, describió la existencia de desigualdades en la mortalidad por clase social en Inglaterra utilizando indicadores de efecto.

Estos indicadores pueden expresar tanto la desigualdad absoluta como la relativa. El primer ejemplo de este artículo (no tabulado) incluye la cuantificación de las magnitudes relativa y absoluta del efecto de las desigualdades en la mortalidad materna en el Cono Sur, durante el período comprendido entre 1992 y 1997. Para ello, se calcularon: (a) la razón de tasas de mortalidad entre el país con mayor producto nacional bruto per cápita (PNB) ajustado por el poder adquisitivo de la moneda (PAM), y el país con menor PNB ajustado por PAM, y (b) la diferencia de tasas entre esos mismos países. Los resultados fueron, respectivamente, 4,9 (123/25) y 98 por 100.000 nacidos vivos (123–25). Esto indica que, en el país con peor situación económica, el riesgo de las gestantes de morir durante el parto o puerperio es casi 5 veces mayor que en el país con mejor situación, y que el valor absoluto de esta desigualdad representa 98 muertes maternas más por cada 100.000 nacidos vivos.

El segundo ejemplo (Figura 2) se refiere al efecto absoluto de las desigualdades en la distribución del ingreso sobre la esperanza de vida al nacer en 1998. Para medir este efecto, se ordenaron los países con más de 500.000 habitantes, de acuerdo con el valor del PNB

---

[3] La relación entre los conceptos de efecto e impacto puede homologarse con la que existe entre las nociones de "riesgo relativo" y "riesgo atribuible" tan bien conocidas en el contexto de la epidemiología.

FIGURA 2. **Esperanza de vida al nacer en la Región de las Américas, quintil inferior y superior de producto nacional bruto (PNB) ajustado por poder adquisitivo de la moneda (PAM), 1997.**

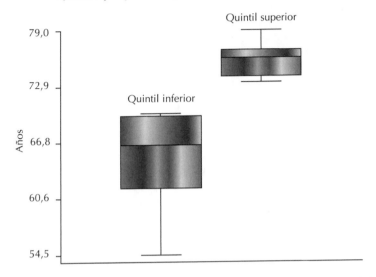

Fuente: Programa Especial de Análisis de Salud (SHA), Organización Panamericana de la Salud (OPS).
Nota: En 1997, la diferencia en la mediana de esperanza de vida al nacer entre los quintiles superior e inferior de ingreso económico en las Américas fue de 9,5 años. En la Región, los más pobres viven cerca de 10 años menos que los más ricos.

corregido, y se calculó la mediana de la esperanza de vida en los quintiles superior e inferior, que fue de 76 años y 66,5 años, respectivamente. En el grupo de países de ingreso más bajo, la esperanza de vida es 9,5 años menor. Esta es, por supuesto, una medida promedio que ilustra el efecto del ingreso sobre la esperanza de vida, pero que puede enmascarar desigualdades, aun de mayor magnitud, que se producen en los países en función del ingreso o de cualquier otro indicador socioeconómico.

La principal objeción a las medidas de efecto presentadas en los ejemplos anteriores, es que solo toman en cuenta los grupos extremos e ignoran los grupos no incluidos en la comparación (7–9). Esta limitación puede superarse mediante el ajuste de modelos de regresión en los cuales uno de los parámetros, o varios, constituyen medidas de efecto que hacen uso de toda la información y no solo de la conte-

nida en grupos escogidos. Esta opción se aplicó en el tercer ejemplo de este estudio (Figura 3), que relaciona la tasa de mortalidad infantil con el acceso a agua potable en varios países de Centroamérica en 1997. La pendiente del modelo de regresión lineal ($\beta = -0,48$) sugiere que por cada 10% de incremento en el acceso a agua potable, la tasa de mortalidad infantil disminuye en 4,8 muertes por cada 1.000 nacidos vivos. Al aplicar estos modelos, es importante prestar atención a la pertinencia del modelo elegido y a la existencia de casos atípicos que pueden distorsionar los parámetros y, por tanto, la estimación de las medidas de desigualdad. En la aplicación de los modelos al estudio de las inequidades con datos agregados, suele ser preferible utilizar el método de estimación de los parámetros basado en mínimos cuadrados ponderados (MCP) en lugar de los mínimos cuadrados ordinarios, debido a las diferencias en los ta-

FIGURA 3. Mortalidad infantil y acceso a agua potable, América Central, 1997.

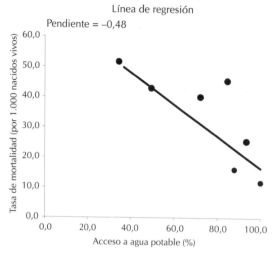

Línea de regresión
Pendiente = –0,48

Fuente: Programa Especial de Análisis de Salud (SHA), Organización Panamericana de la Salud (OPS).

Nota: En América Central, por cada 10% de aumento en el acceso al agua potable, la mortalidad infantil disminuye en 5 muertes por cada 1.000 nacidos vivos en un año.

maños de las unidades; sin embargo, la elección no es automática y debe basarse en los errores estándares de las estimaciones.

IMPACTO DE LAS DESIGUALDADES

Uno de los indicadores de impacto total más conocidos en el campo de la salud es el riesgo atribuible poblacional (RAP), relativo y absoluto. El RAP permite estimar la proporción reducible en la tasa general de morbilidad o mortalidad que se conseguiría si todos los países tuviesen la tasa del grupo de naciones con el nivel socioeconómico más alto. Cuanto más se desvía de cero, mayor es la desigualdad, y mayor su margen de reducción potencial.

En otro de los ejemplos de este estudio (tampoco aparece tabulado) se calculó el RAP asociado a la mortalidad por infección respiratoria aguda (IRA) en niños menores de 5 años. Para ello, se utilizó como referencia la subregión de América del Norte, donde la tasa de mortalidad por IRA de ese grupo de edad era de 0,16

por 1.000 nacidos vivos en 1993, mientras que la tasa total de la Región era de 2,18 por 1.000. El RAP calculado (expresado porcentualmente) fue 92,7%, es decir que si la Región presentase las tasas de América del Norte habría alrededor de 93% menos de defunciones por esta causa para el grupo de edad en cuestión.

Mediante análisis de regresión se calcularon también el índice de desigualdad de la pendiente (IDP) y el índice relativo de desigualdad (IRD) (7–9). Para ello, los países del Caribe con población superior a 150.000 habitantes se ordenaron de acuerdo a su PNB corregido por PAM. El modelo toma como variable dependiente la tasa de mortalidad en niños menores de 5 años, y como variable independiente la proporción relativa acumulada de nacidos vivos. La pendiente (b) del modelo de regresión, ajustado por el método de los MCP, corresponde al IDP y expresa el cambio en la tasa de mortalidad por cada unidad de cambio en la posición relativa en la jerarquía socioeconómica. La tasa de mortalidad en menores de 5 años en 1997 (Figura 4) para el país con PNB corregido más alto fue de 15,3 por 1.000 nacidos vivos, y para el país con PNB más bajo, de 131 por 1.000. La pendiente del modelo fue –142,5 por 1.000, lo que indica que el cambio a un decil superior en la jerarquía socioeconómica en 1997 se acompaña en promedio de una reducción de 14,3 muertes por cada 1.000 niños menores de 5 años. El IRD se obtuvo como el cociente entre el valor de la pendiente β de la regresión y el valor que el modelo predice para la situación económica más alta. El valor así obtenido (10,7) indica que en el país con ingresos más bajos mueren casi 10,7 veces más niños menores de 5 años que en el país con ingresos más altos.

MEDICIÓN DE LAS DESIGUALDADES POR MEDIO DEL COEFICIENTE DE GINI Y DEL ÍNDICE DE CONCENTRACIÓN

El coeficiente de Gini es una medida de desigualdad basada en la curva de Lorenz, con-

FIGURA 4. Mortalidad en menores de 5 años en países del Caribe, 1997.

Línea de regresión

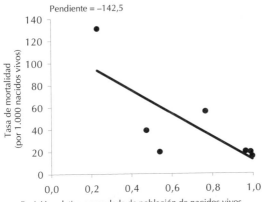

Fuente: Programa Especial de Análisis de Salud (SHA), Organización Panamericana de la Salud (OPS).

Nota: En los países del Caribe que tienen la situación socio-económica más desfavorable, mueren 143 niños menores de 5 años por cada 1.000 más que en los de situación más favorable. Con un índice relativo de desigualdad (IRD) de 10,7, en los países de peor situación mueren casi 11 veces más menores de 5 años que en los de mejor situación.

FIGURA 5. Distribución del ingreso en las Américas, 1996.

Curva de Lorenz

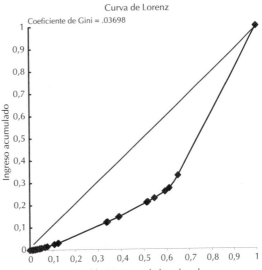

Fuente: Programa Especial de Análisis de Salud (SHA), Organización Panamericana de la Salud (OPS).

Nota: El 30% más rico de la población de las Américas concentra alrededor del 60% del ingreso total.

sistente en una representación gráfica de frecuencias acumuladas que permite comparar la distribución observada de una variable con la distribución uniforme. Esta última está representada por la diagonal con pendiente 1 que pasa por el origen de coordenadas en un sistema de ejes cartesianos. Cuanto mayor es la distancia entre la curva de Lorenz y esta diagonal, mayor es la desigualdad, de modo que la curva proporciona un recurso visual de cuantificación de las desigualdades. El coeficiente de Gini se define como el doble del área comprendida entre la curva de Lorenz y la diagonal de la distribución uniforme.

Un ejemplo clásico es la distribución del ingreso, que en una situación de completa igualdad arroja un valor nulo del coeficiente de Gini, y que en el caso concreto de la Región de las Américas tomó un valor de 0,37 (Figura 5).

La aplicación directa de la curva de Lorenz y el coeficiente de Gini en el contexto de las

desigualdades en salud tiene el inconveniente de que no toma en cuenta la dimensión socioeconómica, pues la población se ordena en función de la variable de salud elegida. Sin embargo, si la población se ordena de menor a mayor ingreso económico, se supera esta desventaja y se obtiene la llamada curva de concentración y su índice de concentración correspondiente.

El índice de concentración de la mortalidad infantil en 1997 en las Américas fue de –0,32, y el de la mortalidad materna en el período de 1992 a 1997 fue de –0,48. En ambos casos, la mortalidad se concentra en los grupos socioeconómicos más pobres. Casi 35% de las defunciones de menores de un año se producen en el quintil más pobre, es decir en el 20% más pobre de la población de nacidos vivos. En el otro extremo, el quintil más rico aporta solo 2% de las muertes maternas.

El índice de concentración se aplicó también al estudio de la distribución del analfabetismo en población femenina en las Américas, en 1995 (Figura 6). Los países de la Región se agruparon y ordenaron de acuerdo con el valor de su PNB per cápita (grupo V: menor ingreso; grupo I: mayor ingreso). La Figura 6 presenta la curva de concentración del analfabetismo en relación con el PNB, y muestra que el 70% del analfabetismo femenino se concentra en el 40% de la población más pobre de las Américas. El índice de concentración es de –0,42.

LA MEDICIÓN DE LAS DESIGUALDADES EN SALUD COMO BASE PARA LA DEFINICIÓN DE POLÍTICAS Y PROGRAMAS

Mediante el uso de indicadores clásicos y de algunas variables de salud elegidas, el presente artículo pone de relieve la existencia de grandes desigualdades en la Región. Este ejercicio descriptivo puede considerarse como un primer paso para la identificación de las inequidades en salud. Hay una gran cantidad de datos agregados disponibles, en especial de mortalidad, morbilidad y otros factores relacionados con la salud, que pueden usarse regularmente en los distintos niveles geopolíticos como base para el análisis de las desigualdades en salud.

La OPS sostiene que la evidencia de una situación de inequidad debe conducir a la ejecución de acciones por parte de los niveles de decisión política, orientadas a disminuirla y, eventualmente, eliminarla. La documentación de las desigualdades en salud es fundamental para definir esas acciones, y, en tal sentido, el fortalecimiento de la capacidad de análisis de los datos que permiten fundamentar la existencia de dichas desigualdades es una condición indispensable. Una vez que se ha instrumentado una intervención específica, los mismos métodos y técnicas de medición y análisis pueden servir para el monitoreo y evaluación de su impacto.

Hay una relación estrecha entre la naturaleza de las intervenciones y las técnicas que se emplean para medir las desigualdades. La metodología y el análisis deben subordinarse a la existencia de un repertorio de acciones factibles y previsibles. Si las acciones previstas suponen el diseño de políticas intersectoriales de alcance poblacional para aumentar al máximo la efectividad, la desigualdad debe documentarse por medio de medidas de impacto; si, por el contrario, las acciones posibles o previstas tienen un carácter intrasectorial y selectivo, las desigualdades deben expresarse por medio de medidas de efecto.

Para la OPS, la búsqueda de equidad en salud no solamente es una cuestión teórica sino un marco concreto para la cooperación técnica con los países, pues la equidad en salud constituye un imperativo para el desarrollo económico regional.

FIGURA 6. **Distribución del analfabetismo femenino en las Américas por grupos de país según ingreso, 1995**

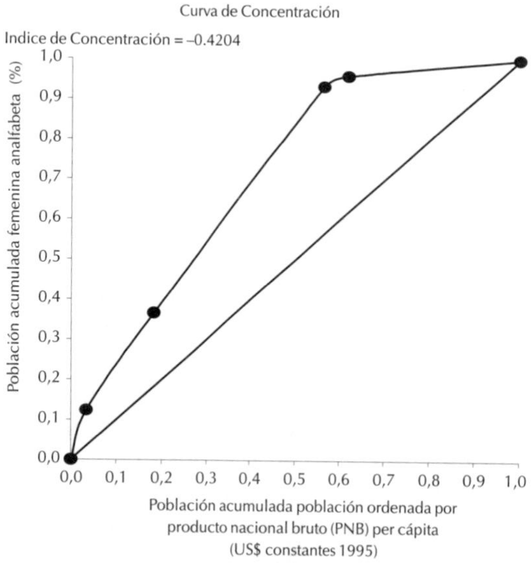

Curva de Concentración

Indice de Concentración = –0.4204

Eje Y: Población acumulada femenina analfabeta (%)

Eje X: Población acumulada población ordenada por producto nacional bruto (PNB) per cápita (US$ constantes 1995)

Fuente: Programa Especial de Análisis de Salud (SHA), Organización Panamericana de la Salud (OPS).

Nota: En 1995, alrededor del 70% del analfabetismo femenino en la Región se concentró en el 40% de la población de ingreso económico más bajo.

REFERENCIAS

1. Organización Panamericana de la Salud. *Las condiciones de salud en las Américas, Edición 1994*, vol. 1. Washington, DC: PAHO; 1994. (Publicación Científica No. 549).

2. Organización Panamericana de la Salud. *Informe Anual del Director 1995. En busca de la equidad.* Washington DC: OPS; 1996. (Documento Oficial No. 277).

3. Organización Panamericana de la Salud. *Informe Anual del Director 1996: Gente sana en entornos saludables.* Washington DC: OPS; 1997. (Documento Oficial No. 283).

4. Organización Panamericana de la Salud. *La salud en las Américas,* edición de 1998, vol. I. Washington DC: OPS; 1998. (Publicación Científica No. 569).

5. Deininger K, Squire L. A new data set measuring income inequality. *The World Bank Economic Review* 1996; 10(3).

6. Alleyne GAO. La salud en el marco de reducción de la pobreza. 5ta. Reunión del Foro Permanente para la Aplicación de la Estrategia de Cooperación al Desarrollo. Lima: Organización Panamericana de la Salud; 1998. (OPS/PER/99.03).

7. Mackenback JP, Kunst AE. Measuring the magnitude of socio-economic inequalities in health: an overview of available measures illustrades with examples from Europe. *Soc Sci Med* 1997; 44(6).

8. Kunst AE, Mackenbach JP. *Measuring socioeconomic inequalities in health. Copenhagen.* WHO Regional Office for Europe; 1994. (EUR/ICP/RPD 416).

9. Wagstaff A, Paci P, van Doorslaer E. On the measurement of inequality in health. *Soc Sci Med* 1991; 33(5).

10. Townsend P, Davidson N. The Black Report. En: Townsend P, Davidson N, Whitehead M (eds). *Inequalities in Health.* London: Penguin Books; 1988.

Noncommunicable Diseases and Risk Factor Surveillance

Sylvia Robles,[1] *Jeanette Vega,*[1] *and Stephen Corber*[1]

INTRODUCTION

The reduction of inequities should be a component of every PAHO technical cooperation program. To be effective in the area of disease control and prevention, the following steps should be undertaken:

1. Identifying and selecting equity-oriented indicators to measure the burden of morbidity and mortality in the Region.
2. Analyzing existing data to identify and quantify the main social inequalities in health (including self-perceived health, morbidity, and mortality) and access to health care, both within and between countries in the Region.
3. Putting information systems in place to monitor health equity as well as trends within and between countries.
4. Developing equity-oriented technical cooperation programs.
5. Conducting periodic evaluations in member countries to assess progress in reducing health inequities as demonstrated by socioeconomic position.

The particular activity that should be undertaken in a given program will depend on the data and technical cooperation that already exists with regard to equity for that program.

MAGNITUDE OF THE PROBLEMS AND TRENDS

Outside of information from the United States and Canada, data from the Region on the relationship between health and the absolute or relative socioeconomic position are scarce, with the possible exception of infant mortality studies (Hollstein et al., 1998; Casas and Dachs, 1998; Paim and Costa, 1993; Victora et al., 1992). Few studies on socioeconomic health inequality, and even fewer that assess time trends or analyze information by causes of adult mortality, have been published. In most Latin American and Caribbean countries, social and economic transformations of the last decades have led to changes in the mortality and morbidity patterns, with an overall decrease in mortality rates and an increase in life expectancy. Noncommunicable diseases (NCDs) now predominate (Murray and Chen, 1993); they account for two-thirds of the mortality in the Region and their proportion is increasing. Fifty percent of these deaths are premature deaths in persons under 65 years of age, which means that they could be prevented or postponed.

[1] Division of Disease Prevention and Control, Pan American Health Organization.

Several behavioral and biological factors have been identified in the scientific literature as risk factors for NCDs, of which the most important are cigarette smoking, a sedentary lifestyle, a high fat diet, obesity, hypercholesterolemia, and hypertension (DHHS, 1991; Stamler, 1987; WHO, 1990). Excessive alcohol consumption is associated with chronic liver disease and is also a major risk factor for disability and death associated with motor vehicle related injuries (DHHS, 1991). Psychosocial factors, including social support, characteristics of the work environment, and depression, have been shown to be related to cardiovascular disease (Marmot, 1982; Berkman, 1982; Rosenman, 1982; Theorell, 1992). Although they are not risk factors in the traditional sense, selected preventive services have proven effective in reducing mortality from cancer of the breast and cervix. There is general agreement that screening by mammography and clinical examination in women 50–69 years of age or older reduces breast cancer mortality (The Canadian Task Force, 1994; US Preventive Services Task Force, 1996), and early detection through PAP smears and other screening methods can decrease mortality from cervical cancer (The Canadian Task Force, 1994; US Preventive Services Task Force, 1996). Similarly, the use of seat belts and helmets has been found to be effective in reducing deaths and disabilities resulting from motor vehicle related injuries (The Canadian Task Force, 1994; US Preventive Services Task Force, 1996). In industrialized countries, improvements in these behavioral risk factors have been associated with marked reductions in the incidence and mortality of the respective NCDs.

Several surveys of NCD risk factors have been conducted in Latin American and the Caribbean, although only Barbados, Colombia, Cuba, and Saint Kitts have conducted these surveys country-wide (Lessa et al., 1996; Martins et al., 1993; Piccini and Victora, 1994; de Lolio et al., 1993a, 1993b; Rego et al., 1990; Llanos and Libman, 1995; Duncan et al., 1993; Litvak et al., 1987; Ordúñez, 1998; Jadue et al., 1999; PAHO, 1997; Ministry of Health of Barbados, 1992). Most studies have been cross-sectional surveys and have not been repeated over time. The exception are the recent efforts in surveillance of tobacco conducted by a few countries, in which increased prevalence of smoking has been described among females and adolescents. Existing evidence suggests that many of these factors are highly prevalent or are becoming highly prevalent in Latin American and Caribbean countries. The prevalence of smoking in adults in those countries has been estimated to range from 30% to 50% in men and from 10% to 30% in women (PAHO, 1992; Lessa et al., 1996; Duncan et al., 1993; de Lolio et al., 1993; Ordúñez et al., 1998; Jadue et al., 1999). Paradoxically, infant malnutrition may coexist with a high prevalence of obesity in some adult populations, reaching as high as 30%–55% in some groups (PAHO, 1998; Foster et al., 1993). The prevalence of hypertension has been estimated to range between 8% and 30% (Lessa et al., 1996; Duncan et al., 1993; Rego et al., 1990; Piccini and Vitora, 1994; de Lolio et al., 1993b; Berrios et al., 1990; Alvarez Perez et al., 1992). Even higher prevalence of hypertension (more than 40%) has been documented in some Caribbean countries (Foster et al., 1993; Ordúñez et al., 1998). High prevalence of hypercholesterolemia (as high as 30%–40%) also has been documented in some areas (Lessa, 1996). The few studies that have quantified physical activity also have documented high prevalence rates of sedentary lifestyle (as high as 50%–90%) (Duncan et al. 1993; Rego et al., 1990; Berrios et al., 1990; Ordúñez et al., 1998; Jadue et al., 1999). Even diabetes, which used to be relatively uncommon in many developing countries, appears to be growing in importance (Vaughan et al., 1989; Phillips and Salmeron, 1992; PAHO, 1998; Llanos and Libman, 1995), with prevalence estimates for Latin American countries generally ranging between 5% and 10% (Llanos and Libman, 1995). Much higher prevalence—as high as 18%—has been documented in some Caribbean countries (Foster et al., 1993). No systematic information on the prevalence of psycho-social factors potentially related to NCDs and injuries exists for the Region.

As with mortality, data related to trends in prevalence and incidence of risk factors according to socioeconomic variables are scarce in the Region, with the exception of some studies conducted in the United States and Canada. In the U.S., studies have shown that most of these risk factors, including perception of health, smoking, physical inactivity, obesity, hypertension, and poor diet, are clustered among individuals in the lower socioeconomic groups. These risks are higher in the most disadvantaged communities, even after adjusting for the individual risk factors, indicating that both individual and contextual characteristics contribute to a person's risk. All of these factors are correlated with an increased risk of mortality over the years (Yen and Kaplan, 1999).

Although some health outcomes are consistently more prevalent in the lower social strata—including, for example, tuberculosis mortality and alcoholism—some of the diseases and associated risk factors evolve over time through social epidemiological transitions. In the first phase of this transition, risk factors are positively associated with socioeconomic position; that is, risk factors are more prevalent in higher socioeconomic groups, although overall incidence of disease may still be low. In the second phase, risk factors become less prevalent in upper social strata, but the incidence of disease increases, while the prevalence of risk factors within the lower social strata remains stable or begins to increase. During this phase, an inverse u-shaped mortality curve might be seen. In the third phase, after the transition is completed, the typical inverse relation between socioeconomic position and risk factor prevalence is observed. Later, due to the time lag between risk exposure and the development of the disease, incidence and premature mortality from NCDs become higher in low socioeconomic groups. For example, the tobacco consumption epidemic may begin in the upper socio-

economic groups, who have the economic resources to purchase cigarettes, and eventually reveal a positive correlation between lung cancer and socioeconomic level. However, over time, persons in lower socioeconomic strata smoke more, while persons in upper socioeconomic groups begin to lower their smoking rates and resort to better technology in the treatment of the disease. Consequently, socioeconomic strata and morbidity/mortality become inversely related.

LIMITATIONS OF THE MEASUREMENTS

In order to measure the strength of the relationship between socioeconomic strata and disease—and thus measure socioeconomic health inequalities—we need to identify and use appropriate indicators, and we must gather sufficient and high-quality data on specific subpopulations.

The Limitations of Measures

Several methods are available for measuring socioeconomic inequalities in health outcomes associated with NCDs. A major methodological issue is the quality of the indicators being used to classify individuals in terms of social position. Another methodological issue concerns the methods used to quantify health inequalities. There is some agreement that in examining social inequalities in health the joint distribution of both health and socioeconomic status should be considered, as should average and dispersion measures. Some of the range measures for mortality and morbidity data for NCDs include comparisons of health between groups at the extremes of the socioeconomic spectrum using rate ratios (RR) or rate differences (RD). The limitation of these measures is that they overlook the intermediate group. Inequalities in health outcomes between the upper and lower socioeconomic groups might, for example, remain unchanged, while inequalities between the intermediate groups and the upper or lower groups might be diminishing or increasing (Wagstaff, 1991).

Several measures of economic inequalities have been developed based on the Lorenz curve, including the Gini coefficient and concentration index. All have the drawback that they measure inequality in relative terms. Other measures have been developed to summarize differences among several groups, taking into account the average level, the differences between groups, and the relative sizes of the groups. One of the most commonly used is the slope index of inequality (SII), which compares the distribution of health outcomes across subgroups; these subgroups are ordered by socioeconomic position by calculating the slope of the (weighted least square) linear regression as a summary measure of health inequality. The result can be interpreted as the rate difference between those at the bottom of the hierarchy and those at the top.

Another issue, especially relevant to NCDs, is that when considering the underlying reasons for the observed differentials in health outcomes in a population, there is a growing consensus that systematic differentials play a prominent role in *exposure to health hazards and risk conditions*. However, depending on the etiologic period, the time interval between exposure and health outcomes can vary, as occurs with changes in mortality associated with changes in prevalence of risk factors for diseases such as cancer, cardiovascular diseases, diabetes, and others. NCDs are characterized by long latency periods between some risk factor exposures and health outcomes, such as with smoking and lung cancer.

Finally, indicators of morbidity may show very different patterns from those in mortality rates, and, therefore, the ranking of countries or communities according to prevalence of diseases will not necessarily match rankings for mortality for those same diseases. Morbidity from NCDs commonly shows much steeper social gradients than mortality, and sex differences are almost always reversed when morbidity is compared to mortality.

Availability and Quality of Data

A serious limitation of all routinely used measurements is that they are based on averages and do not take into account differences among groups—the essence of inequity. Properly designed behavioral risk factor surveys can address this important limitation by collecting and analyzing the information according to different categories of potential inequities (income, education, occupation, gender, race/ethnicity, geography, etc.).

Another limitation of routinely collected data is the fact that information about socioeconomic position for the numerator and denominator of specific rates usually comes from different sources, for example calculating death rates for manual laborers by using death certificates (for the numerator) and census data (for the denominator). This difference can lead to numerator-denominator biases, in which the classification by socioeconomic position indicators varies systematically according to the source. This numerator-denominator problem has been widely discussed in the literature and usually leads to an underestimation of the relationship between socioeconomic position and health risk. The probability of bias can be minimized using aggregated categories (Schkolnikov, 1998) and eliminated using linked registries.

Mortality statistics for NCDs are, on average, fairly reliable over the Americas. However, there are still some countries where coverage and quality of registries need to be improved (PAHO, 1998). A few countries have specific registries for selected problems, for example, cancer registries to provide information about the incidence of malignant neoplasms. One serious limitation of the existing data, however, is that most come from vital statistics registries, which do not always contain information about socioeconomic position, such as income, occupation, and education. When the information is collected, it is usually of poor quality, for example, data on occupational status of the deceased.

The best data for program planning and that can function as an early predictor of the potential benefits of equity-oriented interventions would come from risk factor surveillance through health surveys repeated over time. Experience in some industrialized countries shows that these surveys can give accurate information about the prevalence of risk factors for NCDs, including the differential risks by socioeconomic groups, as well as trends. In these countries, the survey questions have been validated and changes are being monitored over time. A standardized methodology is currently being developed to produce valid and reliable estimates of the prevalence of risk factors in the Region of the Americas. In carrying out behavioral risk factor surveys, questions must be validated to ensure that they are well-understood and will be answered honestly by the respondent in a given environment. Additionally, sampling must be representative, surveyors must be well-trained, and standardized quality control and quality assurance mechanisms at the data collection and data entry levels should be in place. Currently, the lack of standardization of methodologies used across surveys and differences in the information collected makes it difficult to ensure the validity of the results and the comparability among countries and within countries.

INEQUALITIES THAT MAY CONSTITUTE INEQUITIES

Kunst and Mackenbach (1994) argue that an inequality can be measured, while an inequity cannot. However, it does appear possible to measure and study the *perception* of such an inequity in a population or in subgroups of that population.

Evans (1994) uses the term "heterogeneity" and MacIntyre (1997) uses "social patterning" as synonyms for "inequality." These authors clarify that inequalities/heterogeneities/social patterns can refer to differences between groups that are not necessarily socioeconomically determined, but that do have a social

influence, for example, age, gender, marital status, and race/ethnicity. In the framework being presented here, it is assumed that "health inequities" refers to differences in health status related to differences in socioeconomic position (income, education, occupation, race/ethnicity, and gender). Krieger (1997) notes that most measures of socioeconomic position reflect both availability of material and social resources, as well as social status or an individual's rank in a social hierarchy. From this point of view it is important to study and intervene to address the socioeconomic inequities, including gender and race/ethnicity in different geographic settings. The study of gender inequities in NCDs is particularly important, because it is known that some associations between risk factors and disease are not the same in men as in women (Barrett Connor, 1997). Mortality rates associated with NCDs are almost always lower among women than men, and have a lower socioeconomic gradient, but these gender differences are reversed for morbidity and self-perception of disease (women show more morbidity than men, and often show steeper social gradients).

THE INFLUENCE OF DIFFERENT DETERMINANTS

Both the socioeconomic context and health outcomes associated with NCDs can be measured with reference to magnitude and time. It is important to try to clarify the links between health and socioeconomic position, because they are powerful clues about a given society's forms of discrimination which may generate health inequities. Also, in measuring inequities, individual and aggregate-level variables can be used. Aggregate measures for NCDs should mainly be used to compare countries. Mortality comparisons within country, however, should be based on small-area analyses (such as counties) or subpopulations, and survey data is more appropriately analyzed at the individual level.

There is currently little data in the Region about the influence of one determinant on others and about the direct and joint effects of individual and contextual variables. Again, risk factor surveillance can be a key instrument for identifying such influences. The scarce data available have shown some interesting findings. In Valparaiso, Chile, for example, the combined effect of low socioeconomic status and female gender results in higher rates of many risk factors for NCDs.

Additionally, it is important to examine the social context in which a particular risk factor or group of risk factors occurs. Most measurements and interventions currently used for NCD risk factors tend to focus on bringing about behavioral changes in a person, but it is important not to ignore the individual's social environment. The compelling evidence that the lower socioeconomic groups tend to have poorer nutrition, be less physically active in leisure, have greater prevalence of smoking, and have more damaging patterns of alcohol use is only half of the story. It is of critical importance to understand why this is so. The growing literature from qualitative studies on the daily circumstances of people experiencing disadvantages, highlights the greater restrictions on the choice of a healthier lifestyle, due to practical constraints of time, space, and money, as well as psychosocial mechanisms (WHO, 1998). From a methodological perspective, this represents a challenge, since epidemiological studies and surveillance have focused mainly on the individual, and, therefore, assume that personal choice determines behavior. Nonetheless, recent discussions and conceptual approaches have led to new proposals that include both individual and contextual effects—that is, collective characteristics on individual-level outcome measurement and interventions (Diez-Roux, 1998; Van Korff et al., 1992; Hox, 1994). From a public health perspective, this implies that control of risk factors is much harder among the most disadvantaged groups and therefore the interventions should be deliberately tailored towards the worst-off.

HOW TO REDUCE THE GAPS

1. Identifying inequities between and within the Region's countries by implementing monitoring systems.

In the case of routinely collected information, it is crucial to recognize the growing need to supplement vital statistics (such as mortality and birth) and other health data (such as hospital discharge and notification data) with appropriate socioeconomic data that can serve as a foundation for contemporary public health knowledge about patterns and trends of social inequalities in health. This information also can be used to help allocate resources and plan public health interventions at the regional, country, and local levels. Routinely collected mortality data should then be analyzed (at least) by socioeconomic position between countries and ideally for different smaller geographical units within countries. Socioeconomic measures should be included in all health surveys routinely carried out, including risk factor surveys, DHS (Demographic and Health Surveys), and LSMS (Living Standards Measurement Surveys). PAHO could support a line of action that would include validation, standardization, and quality control of risk factor surveys in member countries to facilitate the identification of inequities and create the basis for an ongoing surveillance system for NCDs.

2. Developing a framework to continuously monitor and evaluate progress in countries in achieving health equity for NCDs by taking into account not only the average level of health indicators but also the distribution of health among socioeconomic groups.
3. Collaborating with countries to set health objectives and priorities for NCDs that consider the distribution of health across the population; in other words, set equity targets for the NCD prevention and control health agenda.
4. Working with countries to implement health interventions that address health inequities.

The NCD intervention programs to be developed may not be equally effective in all socioeconomic groups, but efforts should be made to ensure they reach the most disadvantaged. Monitoring of progress should include the extent to which these interventions have been successful in addressing needs and in decreasing health inequities.

5. Reorganizing technical cooperation programs based on an equity-oriented approach.

AN EXAMPLE OF THE USE OF RISK FACTOR SURVEYS TO MONITOR HEALTH INEQUALITIES IN NCDS

The behavioral risk factor survey carried out in Valparaiso, Chile, in 1996 showed several areas of inequalities (Table 1). Surveillance of behavioral risk factors should provide guidance for program planning and maintenance, leading to the reduction of inequities where they exist.

Smoking was highest among males of low socioeconomic status, and overall prevalence was higher among males than females. Among males, no significant differences were observed in the prevalence of obesity, as measured by body mass index, whereas females exhibit higher rates than males. Further, females in the low socioeconomic group exhibit rates significantly higher than females in the middle/high socioeconomic group. Lack of physical activity and the prevalence of hypertension were higher among females than males, and in both groups there was a socioeconomic gradient, with those in the lower end having higher risk. On the other hand, the ratio of total cholesterol to high-density lipoprotein, which indicates the risk of a lipid profile, was higher among the middle/high socioeconomic group among males and females than among the low socioeconomic group. However, when the use of preventive services was analyzed, a higher proportion of males and females in the middle/high socioeconomic group had been tested for cholesterol and glycemia. Further, in spite of the high proportion of women who had had Pap smears, the rate was still lower among those in the low socioeconomic group than in the middle/high group. Further investigation may explain why these differences exist and point to technical cooperation initiatives to address them. Repeated measurement of these risk factors will provide information on trends and on how these differences persist or change.

TABLE 1. Prevalence of risk factors and use of preventive services, by gender and socioeconomic status, Valparaiso, Chile, 1997.

| | Gender and socioeconomic status | | | |
| | Male | | Female | |
	Low (%)	Middle/high (%)	Low (%)	Middle/high (%)
Risk factors				
Regular smoker	50.2	45.5	36.4	34.6
Body mass index ($\geq$25)	62.0	59.5	67.9	60.7
No physical activity	76.5	68.1	97.0	92.1
Hypertension	13.9	10.0	15.7	10.2
Ratio of total cholesterol/ HDL ($\geq$4.5)	47.6	50.0	35.8	39.0
Use of preventive services				
Ever tested for cholesterol	10.9	27.7	18.3	30.5
Ever tested for glycemia	20.4	37.1	43.1	53.6
Ever had a Pap smear	–	–	74.6	81.4

REFERENCES

Alvarez Pérez J, Debs Pino J, Quintana Setién C et al. Comportamiento urbano y rural de factores de riesgo coronario en un estudio comunitario. *Rev Cubana Med Gen Integral* 1992; 8:33–38.

Barbados, Ministry of Health. Barbados Risk Factor Survey; 1992. (Internal report.)

Berkman L. Social network and coronary heart disease. *Adv Cardiol* 1982; 29:37–49.

Berrios X, Jadue L, Zenteno J, et al. Prevalencia de factores de riesgo de enfermedades crónicas: estudio en población general de la región metropolitana. *Rev Med Chile* 1990;118:597–604.

Casas JA, Dachs N. Economic, social and health inequalities in Latin America and the Caribbean; 1998. Printed document.

Casas JA, Dachs JN. Infant mortality and socioeconomic inequalities in the Americas; 1998. Submitted for publication.

de Lolio CM, Pacheco de Souza JM, Hasiak Santo A, Buchalla CM. Prevalência de tabagismo em localidade urbana da região sudeste do Brasil. *Rev Saúde Pública* 1993a; 27:250–61.

de Lolio CM, Rodrigues Pereira JC, Lotufo PA, Pacheco de Souza JM. Hipertensão arterial e possíveis fatores de risco. *Rev Saúde Pública* 1993b; 27:357–62.

Department of Health and Human Services. (1991). *Healthy people 2000: National health promotion and disease prevention objectives.* Washington, DC: Department of Health and Human Services; 1991. Publication No. (PHS)91-50213.

Duncan BB, Schmidt MI, Achutti AC et al. Socioeconomic distribution of noncommunicable disease risk factors in urban Brazil: the case of Pôrto Alegre. *Bull PAHO* 1993; 27:337–349.

Evans RG, Barer ML, Marmor TR (eds). *Why Are Some People Healthy and Others Not? The Determinants of Health of Populations.* New York: de Gruyter; 1994.

Glanz K, Lankenau B, Foerster S, Temple S, Mullis R, Schmid T. Environmental and policy approaches to cardiovascular disease prevention through nutrition: opportunities for state and local action. *Health Educ Quarterly* 1995; 22:512–527.

Hollstein RD, Vega J, Carvajal Y. Desigualdades Sociales y Salud: Nivel Socioeconómico y Mortalidad Infantil en Chile, 1985–1995. *Rev Méd Chile* 1998; 126:333–340.

Kennedy BP, Kawachi I, Glass R and Prothrow-Stih D. Income distribution, socioeconomic status and self rated health in the United States: A multilevel analysis. *BMJ* 1998; 317:917–921.

Krieger N, Williams DR and Moss NE. Measuring Social Class in US Public Health Research. Concepts, Methodologies and Guidelines. *Annu Rev Public Health* 1997; 18:341–78.

Kunst A, Mackenbach J. Measuring socioeconomic inequalities in health. World Health Organization Regional Office for Europe; 1994. (Document).

Jadue L, Vega J, Escobar M, Delgado I, Garrido C, Lastra P, Espejo F, Peruga A. Factores de riesgo para las enfermedades no trasmisibles. Metodología y resultados globales de la encuesta de base del programa CARMEN. *Rev Med Chile*; 1999.

Lessa I, Mendoca GAS, Texeira MTB. Doenças crônicas não-transmissíveis no Brasil: dos fatores de risco ao impacto social. *Bol Of Sanit Panam* 1996; 120:1–25.

Litvak J, Ruiz L, Restrepo H, McAlister A. The growing noncommunicable disease burden, a challenge for the countries of the Americas. *PAHO Bull* 1987; 21:156–171.

Llanos G, Libman I. La diabetes en las Américas. *Bol Oficina Sanit Panam* 1995; 118:1–17.

MacIntyre A. The Black Report and Beyond: What Are the Issues? *Soc Sci Med* 1997; 44;6:723–45.

Markovic N, Bunker CH, Ukoli FA, Kuller LH. John Henrysm and Blood Pressure Among Nigerian Civil Servants. *J Epidemiol Community Health* 1998; 52(3):186–190.

Marmot MG. Psychosocial factors and cardiovascular disease: epidemiological approaches. *Europ H J* 1988;9:690–697.

Martins IS, Coelho LT, Mazzilli RN et al. Doenças cardiovasculares ateroscleróticas, dislipidemias, hipertensão, obesidade e diabetes melito em populaçao da área metropolitana da região sudeste do Brasil. I-Metodología da pesquisa. *Rev Saúde Pública* 1993; 27:250–61.

Murray C, Chen L. In Search of a Contemporary Theory for Understanding Mortality Change. *Soc Sci Med* 1993; 36(2):143–155.

Nobak M, Pikhart H, Hertzman C, Rose R, Marmot M. Socioeconomic Factors, Perceived Control and Self-reported Health in Russia. A Cross-sectional Survey. *Soc Sci Med* 1998; 47(2):269–279.

Ordúñez PO, Espinosa A, Cooper R, Kaufman J, Nieto J. Hypertension in Cuba: evidence of narrow black-white difference. *J Hum Hypertens* 1998; 12: 111–116.

Pan American Health Organization. *Annual Report of the Director, 1998: Information for Health.* Washington, DC: PAHO; 1999. (Official Document No. 293).

Pan American Health Organization. Report Risk Factor Survey in St. Vincent. PAHO, Caribbean Program Coordination; 1997. (Document).

Pan American Health Organization. *Health in the Americas, 1998 Edition.* vol. 1. Washington, DC: PAHO; 1998. (Scientific Publication No. 569).

Pan American Health Organization. *Tobacco or health: Status in the Americas.* Washington, DC: PAHO; 1992. (Scientific Publication No. 536).

Paim J, Costa MC. Decline and Unevenness of Infant Mortality in Salvador, Brazil, 1980–1988. *Bol Of Sanit Panam* 1993; 27(1):1–14.

Phillips M, Salmeron J. Diabetes in Mexico—A serious and growing problem. *World Health Stat Quart* 1992; 45:338–346.

Piccini RX, Vitora CG. Hipertensão arterial sistêmica em área urbana no sul do Brasil: prevalência e fatores de risco *Rev Saúde Pública* 1994; 28:261–267.

Rego RA, Berardo FAN, Rodrigues SR, et al. Fatores de risco para doenças crônicas não-transmissíveis: inquérito domiciliar no municio de São Paulo, Brasil. Metodología e resultados preliminares. *Rev Saúde Pública* 1990; 24:277–285.

Robles S, White F, Peruga A. Trends in Cervical Cancer Mortality in the Americas. *Bol Of Sanit Panam* 1996; 30(4):290–301.

Rosenman RH. Role of type A behavior in the pathogenesis and prognosis of coronary heart disease. *Adv Cardiol* 1982; 29:77–84.

Shkolnikov VM, Leon DA, Adamets S, Andreev E and Deev A. Educational Level and Adult Mortality in Russia: An Analysis of Routine Data 1979 to 1994. *Soc Sci Med* 1998; 47(3):357–69.

Stamler J. Epidemiology, established major risk factors, and the primary prevention of coronary heart disease. In: Parmley WW, Chatterjee K (eds). *Cardiology* Vol. 2. Philadelphia: Lippincott; 1987.

The Canadian Task Force on the Periodic Health Examination. The Canadian Guide to Clinical Preventive Health Care. Ottawa, Canada: Canada Communication Group; 1994.

Theorell T. The psychosocial environment, stress, and coronary heart disease. In: Marmot M, Elliot P (eds.). *Coronary heart disease: from etiology to public health*. New York: Oxford University Press; 1992.

United States Department of Health and Human Services. *The health benefits of smoking cessation: A Report of the Surgeon General*. Rockville: U.S. Department of Health and Human Services, Public Health Service, Centers for Disease Control, Center for Chronic Disease Prevention and Health Promotion, Office on Smoking and Health; 1990. (DHHS Publication No. CDC 90-8416).

US Preventive Services Task Force. *Guide to clinical preventive services: report of the U.S. Preventive Services Task Force*. 2nd ed. Baltimore: Williams and Wilkins; 1996.

Vaughan P, Gilson L, Mills A. Diabetes in developing countries: its importance for public health. *Health Policy and Planning* 1989; 4:97–109.

Victora C, Barros F, Hutley S, Teixeira AM, Vaughan JP. Early childhood mortality in a Brazilian cohort: The roles of birthweight and socioeconomic status. *Intern J Epidemiol* 1992; 21:359–65.

Wagstaff A, Paci P, van Doorslaer E. On the measurement of inequalities in health. *Soc Sci Med* 1991; 33(5):545–57.

Whitehead M. The health divide. In: Townsend P, Whitehead M, and Davidson N (eds.). *Inequalities in Health. The Black Report and the Health Divide*. London: Penguin; 1992.

World Health Organization. Diet, nutrition, and the prevention of chronic diseases. Geneva: WHO; 1990. (Technical Report Series No. 797.)

Winkleby MA, Jatulis DE, Frank E, Fortmann SP. Socioeconomic status and health: How education, income, and occupation contribute to risk factors for cardiovascular disease. *Am J Public Health* 1992; 82(6):816–820.

Yen IH, Kaplan G. Neighborhood social environment and risk of death: Multilevel evidence from the Alameda County study. *American Journal of Epidemiology* 1999; 149(10):898–906.

HEALTH EQUITY AND MATERNAL MORTALITY

Ernesto Pate,[1] Carol Collado,[1] and Jose Antonio Solís[1]

INTRODUCTION

Each year, 600,000 women between the ages of 15 and 45 die in the world from complications arising from pregnancy and childbirth. And for every woman who dies, many more suffer morbidity that can affect them for the rest of their lives. The tragedy is that these women die not from disease, but during the normal life-enhancing process of procreation. What is worse is the fact that most of these deaths could be avoided if preventive measures were taken and adequate care were available.

Maternal mortality is not merely a "health disadvantage," it is a "social disadvantage." Health, social, and economic interventions are most effective when they are implemented simultaneously. Since the 1940s, maternal deaths in the developed world have become increasingly rare. Not so in developing areas, where persistently high maternal mortality levels are symptomatic of a pervasive neglect of women's most fundamental human rights, a neglect that is most acutely suffered by the poor, the disadvantaged, and the powerless. The level of maternal mortality reflects women's place in society, as well as their access to social health and nutrition services and economic opportunities.

Ultimately, maternal death is a tragedy for individual women, families, and their communities. The impact of maternal death is felt by the whole family and rebounds across the generations. The complications that cause the death and disability of mothers also damage the infants they carry. The poor health and lack of care that contribute to the death of women in pregnancy and childbirth also compromise the health and survival of the infants and children they leave behind. It affects the family's well-being and that group's potential to contribute to the development of the community. It is estimated that nearly two-thirds of the eight million infant deaths that occur each year result largely from poor maternal health and hygiene, inadequate care, inefficient delivery management, and lack of essential care of the newborn. The social costs to the immediate family group are compounded with economic costs to the health care system and missed development opportunities.

MATERNAL MORTALITY IN THE REGION OF THE AMERICAS

What Is a Maternal Death?

A maternal death, according to the *International Statistical Classification of Diseases and Related Health Problems, Tenth Revision* (ICD-10), is the death of a woman who was preg-

[1]Division of Health Promotion and Protection, Pan American Health Organization.

nant at the time of death or had recently been so, and whose death was related directly or indirectly to the pregnancy. Direct maternal deaths are those resulting from complications of pregnancy occurring in the prenatal period, during labor and childbirth, or within 42 days following termination of the pregnancy. Recently, the following has been added: ". . . irrespective of the duration and site of the pregnancy, from any cause related or aggravated by the pregnancy or its management but not from accidental or incidental causes." Further, maternal deaths are to be reported in two groups: (a) direct obstetric deaths and (b) indirect obstetric deaths. ICD-10 also recognizes late maternal deaths as those deaths occurring up to one year after the termination of the pregnancy. However, the applications of these changes in definition are not uniform among countries, even in those with good registration systems.

Why Do Women Die?

Globally, approximately 80% of all maternal deaths are the direct result of complications arising during pregnancy, delivery, or the puerperium. It should be noted, however, that there is under-reporting of deaths and their causes, and the available databases are weak. The most commonly registered clinical causes of death in Latin America and the Caribbean are characterized below:

- *Hemorrhage, especially postpartum,* which results in 20% of maternal deaths, is unpredictable, sudden in onset and swift to kill. It can lead to death very rapidly in the absence of appropriate and prompt lifesaving care.
- *Hypertensive disorders of pregnancy,* particularly eclampsia (convulsions), result in some 20% of all maternal deaths.
- *Abortion complications* cause 16% of maternal deaths. Laws should ensure the availability of services for the management of abortion complications and post-abortion

care. Where abortion is legal, safe pregnancy termination should be made available. National policy can discourage the use of unsafe abortion by providing protection against unwanted pregnancy and establishing national health campaigns to raise awareness of the risks of unsafe abortion and to show how to recognize and seek treatment for abortion complications.
- *Complications of pregnancy,* responsible for 14% of maternal deaths, include puerperal infections, often the consequence of poor hygiene during delivery or untreated STIs, and prolonged or obstructed labor, caused by cephalopelvic disproportion or by an abnormal positioning of the fetus.

Many of the above medical problems are aggravated by chronic or residual conditions. Of these indirect contributors to death, one of the most significant is anemia, which also is thought to underlie a substantial proportion of direct deaths (particularly those caused by hemorrhage and sepsis), as well as contribute to death by cardiovascular arrest.

The Health Disadvantage

Within the above-mentioned clinical causes, there is a clear relationship between the population and the health care system. A good number of the deaths could have been prevented through timely quality care. Examples of this would be: careful monitoring during pregnancy and the post-partum period; treatment with relatively simple measures and drugs; access to specific services such as family planning; attendance at birth by trained personnel; and attention to cultural and ethnic practices that exacerbate or potentiate problems.

Approximately two-thirds of all pregnant women in Latin America and the Caribbean deliver with the help of skilled attendants. Many women, however, are assisted only by relatives or traditional birth attendants, and many deliver alone. Providing birthing women with a skilled attendant who is able to prevent, detect, and manage the major obstetric complications and who has the equipment, drugs, and supplies to treat them effectively is considered to be the single most important factor in preventing maternal deaths. Data from Peru shows that trained personnel attend only 16% of deliveries by women within the lowest quartile of household assets. In comparison, trained personnel deliver 92% of women within the highest quartile of household assets (see Figure 7 in the chapter titled "Health Disparities in Latin America and the Caribbean: The Role of Social and Economic Determinants," which appears in Part 1 of this publication).

The lack of access to and utilization of quality obstetric services is a crucial factor leading to high maternal mortality. Although an estimated 15% of pregnant women will experience life-threatening complications that require emergency care, there are virtually no data on the proportion of women with access to such care. As many as 40% of pregnancies are likely to require some form of special care.

The Social Disadvantage

While the above sections speak to the clinical causes of maternal mortality, there also are a number of social disadvantages leading these women along a death march. These involve many contextual factors such as socioeconomic factors, cultural and ethnically based belief systems and practices, and geographical barriers, to name a few.

Some women's low social status limits their access to economic resources, basic health resources, and educational resources, among others. It also affects their ability to make decisions related to their health and nutritional needs and to seek assistance.

Many other factors underlie the medical causes of maternal mortality, such as poverty, low income, poor nutrition, excessive physical work, lack of decision-making power, and cultural beliefs. The common pathway for most of these factors is poor access to care.

EVIDENCE IN MATERNAL MORTALITY MEASUREMENT

Trends in Maternal Mortality in Latin America and the Caribbean

Longitudinal data from PAHO from 1960 to 1980 shows that the maternal mortality ratios in all countries have fallen, but the rate of decline has been slow in the less developed countries. There are still vast differences between countries in the Region; more than 10 countries continue to suffer maternal mortality ratios greater than 100 per 100,000 live births (see Figure 1).

Measures of Maternal Mortality

There are three main measures of maternal mortality: the maternal mortality ratio, the maternal mortality rate, and the lifetime risk of maternal death.

- The *maternal mortality ratio* represents the obstetric risk associated with each pregnancy, described as the number of maternal deaths per 100,000 live births during a one year period. Although it has traditionally been called a rate, this is actually a ratio and is now usually called such by researchers.
- The *maternal mortality rate* measures both the obstetric risk and the frequency with which women are exposed to this risk, and is calculated as the number of maternal deaths per 100,000 women of reproductive age (usually 15–49 years) during a given period.
- The *lifetime risk of maternal death* takes into account both the probability of becoming pregnant and the probability of dying as a result of that pregnancy, accumulated across a woman's reproductive years. The lifetime risk is calculated using the maternal mortality ratio and the total fertility rate, increased by 25% to allow for pregnancy wastage.

FIGURE 1. Maternal mortality per 100,000 live births, selected countries in the Americas, 1960, 1970, 1980, and circa 1984.

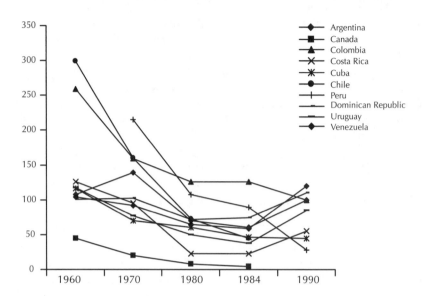

Because the term "ratio" and "rate" are often used interchangeably, for the sake of clarity it is essential to specify the denominator used when referring to either of the first two measures of maternal mortality.

The setting where the problem of maternal mortality is most acute is precisely that in which it is least likely to be accurately measured. Of the 600,000 maternal deaths that occur yearly around the world, most occur in developing countries. If we focus on the Region of the Americas, in Canada the maternal mortality ratio averages about 4 maternal deaths per 100,000 live births (1995); in contrast, in Latin America and the Caribbean the ratio is nearly 20 times higher. Because the maternal mortality ratio represents a measure of the obstetric risk every time a woman becomes pregnant, the risk of maternal death is magnified in areas where women have many pregnancies in their lifetime.

In developing countries, 1 woman in 12 may die of pregnancy-related causes, compared with 1 in 4,000 in industrialized countries. The discrepancy between these two figures not only represents one of the starkest and most telling differentials in development, but also reflects the huge differences in national commitment between different developing countries.

In the Region of the Americas, a woman's lifetime risk of dying during pregnancy and childbirth ranges from 1:17 (Haiti), to 1:510 (Panama), to 1:3,700 (USA), and to 1:7,000 (Canada). These disparities can be largely explained by poor access to quality care.

Measurement Limitations

As experience with implementing "safe motherhood" programs[2] has grown, it has become increasingly clear that the traditional indicator of maternal health status—the ma-

---

[2] The safe motherhood initiative was founded at an international conference in Nairobi in 1987 to address the high maternal mortality seen in developing countries. Over the past decade of advocacy and action for safe motherhood, a broad range of needed interventions has been mapped out by the many partners working in this area, including governments, multilateral and bilateral funding agencies, technical support agencies, NGO's, and other interested parties. However, the interventions iden-

ternal mortality ratio—is not an appropriate indicator for monitoring progress in the short term. Maternal mortality ratios are inappropriate for short-term monitoring:

- The maternal mortality ratio is not sensitive to changes in the delivery of care and, therefore, is not very useful as a monitoring tool.
- Few developing countries have the sophisticated and comprehensive systems of vital registration needed to accurately monitor levels of maternal mortality. In such circumstances, household surveys have to be used to estimate maternal mortality.
- Maternal deaths are relatively rare events even where maternal mortality is high. Thus, all household survey techniques are subject to wide margins of error and are very expensive to implement.
- The simple measurement tools developed in recent years, such as the sisterhood method, are not appropriate for regular monitoring purposes because they provide data relating to a point some time in the past.

Surveillance Issues

As a result of the measurement limitations and for other technical reasons, most maternal mortality reduction programs now rely on process indicators for regular program monitoring. Such process indicators can include the number and distribution of essential obstetric-care services, the proportion of deliveries attended by skilled health care providers or occurring in institutional settings, or the rates of operative delivery and institutional case fatality rates.

Guidelines have been developed to assist countries in gathering, analyzing, and interpreting such indicators. These process indicators describe the major pathway to reducing maternal mortality in terms of access to essential obstetric care, appropriate utilization of such services, and some aspects of quality of care. An important advantage of these measures is that they are not only relevant for monitoring progress, but also permit policy-makers and planners to better target interventions to reduce maternal mortality and morbidity. They often are derived from routine data or as part of program implementation, thus limiting data collection costs.

While process indicators such as these are useful for monitoring programs, more detailed investigation is needed to diagnose the underlying causes of maternal mortality and to identify ways of dealing with them.

Maternal mortality is under-reported worldwide, and most of the figures reported for developing countries are estimates. Surveys done in Latin America and the Caribbean show that we should multiply our reported rates by a factor between 1.5 and 2.3.

In Argentina in 1995, Elida Marconi used a systematic process to reduce misclassification by matching death certificates to clinical records, and found that the extent of misclassification for the country as a whole was 53%. Consequently, official estimates of maternal mortality should be adjusted by a factor of 1.53 to correct for errors in classification.

To describe the Brazil experience, Ruy Lurentis compared the official maternal mortality ratio of 44 per 100,000 live births to the study's finding, a ratio of 99.6 per 100,000 live births. This meant that there was an under-reporting of 65.9%, which requires an adjustment factor of 2.26 when all factors are considered.

Recent research has highlighted the extent of under-reporting and misclassification of maternal deaths, even in countries with good vital registration (Atrash et al., 1995). Research in the USA, which used six different sources in addition to published vital records to iden-

---

tified have not always been implemented systematically or comprehensively, and although there have been some successful examples, global progress has been slow.

The inter-ministerial meeting held in Lima in 1998 looked at progress in this area since 1990 and stated that the reduction in maternal mortality has reached a plateau. This has resulted in the formation of the inter agency task force comprised of PAHO, UNFPA, UNICEF, UNIFEM, USAID, The World Bank, and IADB to coordinate activities in this area.

tify deaths related to pregnancy, also detected significant under-reporting. No single source of information identified all maternal deaths.

In some countries, there is a tendency to report higher levels of maternal mortality where there is an expectation of receiving funding for program activities, and to report lower levels when it was necessary to demonstrate success. These tendencies aggravate the inaccurate reporting.

DALYs (Disability Adjusted Life Years) measures are a time-based indicator of health outcome that forms a composite measure of the overall burden of disease due to losses from premature death and non-fatal disability. DALYs are the measurement unit for the global burden of disease study (GBD); they have been designed to assist with cost effectiveness analysis and are used as a tool for priority setting. This single outcome measure has limitations because only a restricted number of dimensions of health care can be taken into account. Some experts have expressed concerns that the methodology may reinforce a medical model of health care and narrow vertical approaches. DALYs should not be used as the only tool for prioritization or resource allocation. Recommendations are currently being developed to enable DALYs to better capture the burden of reproductive ill health and will be used in the revision of the GBD study planned for 2000.

A CLOSER LOOK AT INEQUITIES

Differences between Men and Women

Health expectancies make it possible to specify inequities between social groups, regions in a country, and sexes. It is increasingly clear that a very strong relationship exists between short life expectancy and amount of morbidity (Robine et al., 1999). Although this relationship has been demonstrated by data in developed countries, no such calculations have been made for Latin American and Caribbean countries. Data from Latin America

and the Caribbean, however, show a high mortality and morbidity among females due to reproductive health causes.

Most studies indicate that life expectancy and positive health expectancy are higher for females than for males, but the proportion of morbidity-free years to total life expectancy is slightly lower for females. The difference in life expectancy between the sexes is reduced when an estimate of health expectancy is produced. Results from studies using data from repeated wave surveys have suggested that the greater proportion of years lived with disability or handicap by women may be explained by the longer survival of women after the development of these problems.

Life expectancy in Latin America and the Caribbean has been increasing in all countries over the past decade, but this increase is lower in countries with high maternal mortality, and is also closely linked to education.

Socioeconomic Differences

Socioeconomic differences have been studied for nine countries. All but one of the studies has demonstrated that social inequalities in health are much greater than has been shown by differential mortality. Not only are the poorest and the least educated people shorter-lived, but they also experience a greater part of their lives with disability or handicap. This was first observed in Canada: the difference in life expectancy between the richest 20% and the poorest 20% in the community was 6.3 years, but increased to 14.3 years for disability-free life expectancy.

Finnish and Dutch studies have demonstrated socioeconomic inequalities by means of calculations using several educational levels, and found that the higher the educational level, the higher both life expectancy and positive health expectancy. Kennedy et al. (1996) have shown that race along with other socioeconomic differences are good predictors of excess mortality. Calculations comparing different ethnic groups in the USA show much lower life expectancies and disability-free life expectancies for black people than for Asian people as compared to whites.

Studies show that socioeconomic differences, including education and race, are closely related to maternal mortality. Although this data is not readily available for Latin America and the Caribbean, infant mortality parallels maternal mortality trends in the region, and some data exist in this area.

Data from Brazil shows a six-fold difference in infant mortality between families in the highest and the lowest income groups, and this difference holds true even for data collected ten years apart (see Figure 4 in the chapter "Health Disparities in Latin America and the Caribbean: The Role of Social and Economic Determinants," which appears in Part 1 of this publication).

Geographical Comparisons within Countries

Rural Versus Urban Disparities

Data from Guatemala shows that areas with high percentages of indigenous people have higher maternal mortality than other areas. Associated with this increased mortality is lower life expectancy among females, lower availability of water, lower literacy, and lower spending on health services. In general in Latin America and the Caribbean, analyses show that most maternal deaths occur in rural areas. In Guatemala, there are 0.3 hospital beds per 10,000 people in the rural population, compared to 1.3 hospital beds per 10,000 people in the urban population. Such disparities in the distribution of resources can cause inequities in health outcomes such as mortality. There is little direct data reporting on rural/urban differences for most of the countries in LAC. This is in itself an inequity as it prevents and delays action being taken to reach the underserved populations (see Figures 2–6).

Factors resulting in an increased risk of maternal morbidity and mortality also affect the fetus and young child, and frequently re-

FIGURE 2. Socioeconomic stratification of departments according to percentages of the gross domestic product, indigenous population, and rural inhabitants, Guatemala, 1998.

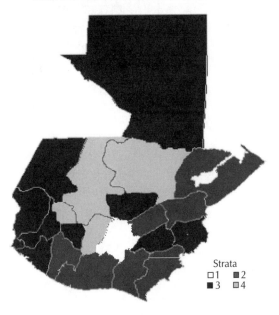

sult in low birthweight and, later, stunting in children. Using low birthweight and stunting in children as indirect measures of inequalities in maternal mortality risk factors, we can further demonstrate rural/urban differences in Latin American and Caribbean countries. Data from these countries show an almost two-fold increase in low birthweight and stunting in children from rural areas. At the same time, there has been a 68% decline in infant mortality rates in low birthweight babies born to wealthy parents over a ten-year period in Brazil, but only a 36% decline in infant mortality in low birthweight babies born to poor parents (see Figures 7 and 8).

Maternal Mortality and Educational Levels

Maternal mortality is greatest among women with the lowest educational level, 30%–50% of whom never arrive at the health facilities. This is especially true in rural areas.

FIGURE 3. Female life expectancy, according to socioeconomic group, Guatemala.

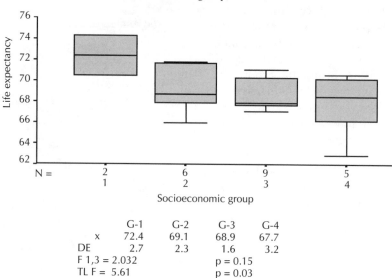

	G-1	G-2	G-3	G-4
x	72.4	69.1	68.9	67.7
DE	2.7	2.3	1.6	3.2
F 1,3 = 2.032			p = 0.15	
TL F = 5.61			p = 0.03	

FIGURE 4. Available water according to socioeconomic group, Guatemala.

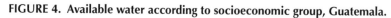

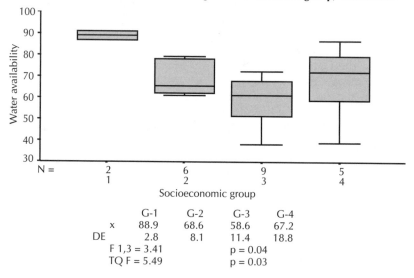

	G-1	G-2	G-3	G-4
x	88.9	68.6	58.6	67.2
DE	2.8	8.1	11.4	18.8
F 1,3 = 3.41			p = 0.04	
TQ F = 5.49			p = 0.03	

FIGURE 5. Female illiteracy according to socioeconomic group, Guatemala.

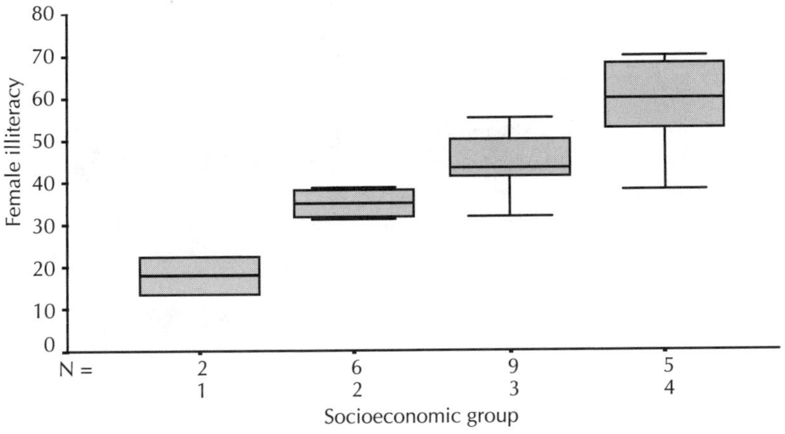

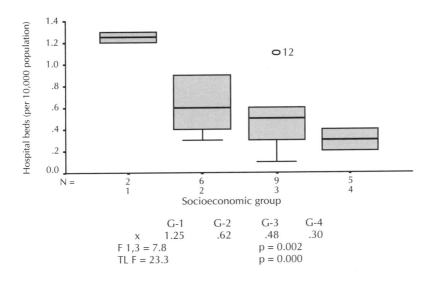

	G-1	G-2	G-3	G-4
x	18.0	34.9	44.3	57.7
DE	6.3	3.1	7.8	12.9

F 1,3 = 13.3   p = 0.000
FTL = 36.6   p = 0.000

FIGURE 6. Distribution of hospital beds per 10,000 population according to socioeconomic group, Guatemala.

	G-1	G-2	G-3	G-4
x	1.25	.62	.48	.30

F 1,3 = 7.8   p = 0.002
TL F = 23.3   p = 0.000

FIGURE 7. Percent reductions in infant mortality rates in Pelotas, Southern Brazil, between 1982 and 1993, by income group and birthweight.

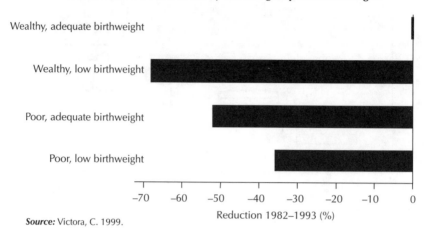

Source: Victora, C. 1999.

FIGURE 8. Percentage of stunting in children below 5 years of age, according to urban or rural area, selected countries, Latin America and the Caribbean, early to middle 1990s.

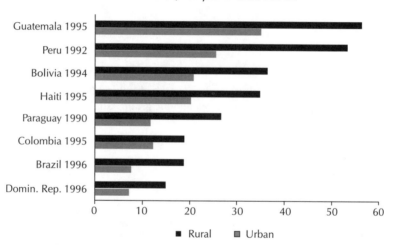

Source: Demographic and Health Surveys, DHS.

Data from Chile shows that life expectancy is lowest for women with no education and increases rapidly as the years of schooling increase. Further, this difference has widened over the past ten years. In 1996 the life expectancy for a 20-year-old woman with no education was 53 years, compared to 72 years for a woman with 13 or more years of schooling— a striking difference of 19 years of life expectancy (see Figure 10 in the chapter titled "Health Disparities in Latin America and the Caribbean: The Role of Social and Economic Determinants," included elsewhere in this publication).

Not only do race and education levels affect maternal mortality and life expectancy, but they also affect the mortality and morbidity of the children. A recent study from Brazil by Pinto da Cunha (1997) on infant mortality showed that infant mortality was highest for infants of black mothers, decreased for infants of mulatto and dark mothers, and was lowest for infants of white mothers, among mothers with no formal education. This trend persisted consistently as years of schooling in the mothers increased (see Figure 14 in the chapter titled "Health Disparities in Latin America and the Caribbean: The Role of Social and Economic Determinants," included elsewhere in this publication).

Economic Inequities

As described elsewhere in this publication, Latin America is the region with greatest social and economic disparities. In this Region, 60% of the national income is earned by the richest 20% of the population (see Figure 9).

The introduction of extensive economic adjustment and reform programs in the Region, with policies of free trade, currency liberalization, and reduction of government expenditures, has resulted in moderate economic growth since 1990. These changes have not had any significant impact on levels of poverty or on employment. Data show that in Latin America and the Caribbean, the percentage of the population living in absolute poverty has increased, widening the gap between the urban and rural populations. This Region demonstrates a model of growth without distribution (see Figures 10 and 11).

Income Disparities

Reduction of mortality in infants under 1 year old is strongly associated with an increase in total available resources in the society. The general data for the Americas in 1996 demonstrates that lower national infant mortality rates correlate with the increase in per capita income adjusted for purchasing power parity.

However, in countries in which per capita income adjusted for purchasing power parity falls below $4,000, the disparities in the internal distribution of income seem to be poorly associated with the level of mortality. In these societies, it seems that the total amount of resources is more a determinant of the health status of the population than the internal distribution of these resources. Although subnational groups with more or less per capita income may exist, the national health status is more associated with the total amount of available resources.

In general, per capita income greatly influences the distribution and utilization of health care resources in Latin America and the Caribbean (see Figure 12 for data for Bolivia and Peru). This is clearly demonstrated by data from Mexico showing that as per capita income increases the percentage of hospital deliveries, and number of physicians and beds per inhabitant increases exponentially (Lozano et al., 1999) (see Figure 7 in the chapter titled "Health Disparities in Latin America and the Caribbean: The Role of Social and Economic Determinants," included elsewhere in this publication).

FIGURE 9. Percent of national income by income quartiles, selected regions of the world.

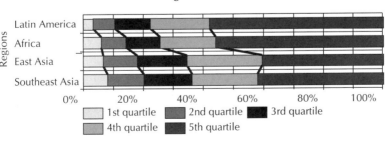

FIGURE 10. People living in extreme poverty (in thousands), 19 countries.

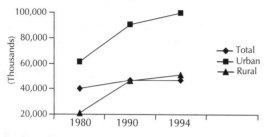

FIGURE 12. Inequity in delivery assistance by income quartiles, Bolivia and Peru.

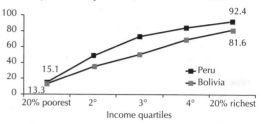

Source: World Bank, 1998 (unpublished).

In countries whose per capita income adjusted for purchasing power parity falls above the $4,000 threshold, the absolute level of wealth or available resources no longer explains differences in health status. In these countries the infant mortality rate and maternal mortality ratio tend to be higher in the countries with higher income disparities, measured as the ratio of the income of the highest 20% of the population and the income of the lowest 20%. Countries with the highest income disparities have infant mortality rates up to three times higher than those with less disparity.

These examples demonstrate that a country's overall wealth is not, in itself, the most important determinant of maternal mortality. There are examples of countries with modest levels of GNP and with low income disparities that are coupled with low maternal mortality.

FIGURE 11. Poverty rates in 19 countries in Latin America.

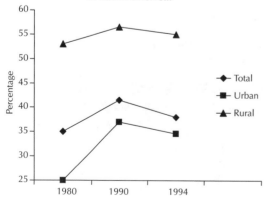

Clearly, in situations where the level of wealth available to the majority of the population is low and the income disparity is significant, access to quality care will be affected and maternal mortality and morbidity will be high.

Inequity among Countries in Latin America and the Caribbean

As demonstrated by maternal mortality ratios, the disparities among countries in the Americas are made even more manifest by comparing the ratio of national maternal mortality rates with the regional minimum rate. There is a 14-fold difference in infant mortality rates between the Region's countries with the lowest infant mortality rates and those with the highest rates. If a similar comparison is carried out for maternal mortality we will see a greater than 100-fold difference in two countries and a 20-fold difference in more than half of the countries in Latin America and the Caribbean. These enormous differences in maternal mortality have much to do with inaccessibility to quality health care. It is important to stress that while a large proportion of infant deaths are due to environmentally related conditions—diarrheal diseases, acute respiratory infections, and malnutrition—maternal mortality is almost wholly attributable to a lack of or poor quality prenatal and perinatal care (see Figure 3 in the chapter titled "Health Disparities in Latin America and the Caribbean: The Role of Social and Economic Determinants," included elsewhere in this volume).

Actions to Reduce Maternal Mortality

The historical record demonstrates that rapid reductions in levels of maternal mortality can be achieved when key interventions are in place. Ten years of implementing safe motherhood programs has shown that we can advance safe motherhood through:

- improving human rights;
- empowering women and ensuring choice;
- acknowledging that safe motherhood is a vital social and economic investment;
- delaying first birth;
- planning ahead to deal with pregnancy risks since every pregnancy faces risks;
- ensuring skilled attendants at each delivery (this requires national policies favoring professionals with midwifery skills for all births, coupled with standards for quality of care);
- improving access to maternal services by establishing community-based maternal health care systems comprising prenatal, delivery, and postpartum care and a system of referral to a higher level of care when obstetric complications arise; and
- preventing unwanted pregnancy and addressing unsafe abortions.

Countries vary enormously in terms of the situations and challenges they face and in terms of their capacity to address these challenges. However, experience has demonstrated that several features are common to successful efforts to address maternal mortality, such as carrying out:

- coordinated efforts over the long term;
- actions within families and communities, and in society at large;
- actions at the legal and policy level and in health systems;
- interactions among the interventions in these areas, which are critical for reducing maternal mortality and for building and supporting momentum for change; and
- political will to implement change.

There will be a need to support:

- a social, economic, and legislative environment that will enable women to obtain health care and overcome the multiple barriers that reduce their access to this care;
- policies ensuring that all couples and individuals have access to good quality, client-oriented, and confidential family planning information and services that offer a wide choice of effective contraceptive methods—policies should address the regulatory, social efforts to offset economic and cultural factors that limit women's control over sexuality and reproduction;
- services that assign health workers trained in midwifery to community-based health facilities, thus reducing barriers to access due to distance, lack of transport, and costs of services;
- health care services developed with protocols and statutes for providing routine maternal care and managing obstetric complications at each level of the health system; and
- decentralized services that are as close to people's homes as possible—particularly in rural and remote areas, facilities must have supplies, equipment, and trained staff.

CONCLUSIONS

Maternal Mortality is an Area of Significant Inequity in Health in Latin America and the Caribbean

If we are to help reduce inequity we must clearly identify the unfair disparities in health that occur in our countries and apply those technologies that reduce those disparities. In the case of maternal mortality, the disparities are multi-faceted and complex. Many factors are outside of the control of the health sector; some are supply-driven while others are demand-driven.

Data from the Region shows that we need to increase access to quality care. Research has shown that accessibility does not necessarily imply usage. The motivation of the socially disadvantaged to make use of services that are theoretically accessible may not be the same as for the more fortunate groups, even apart from the differences in transactional costs. We initially thought that the socially disadvantaged were more resistant to changing risk behaviors; we now know this is not the case.

Current research shows that issues of respect, confidentiality, auditory and visual privacy in the service areas, dialogue, and sharing of information are as important as the medical therapy being provided in encouraging utilization of resources.

Improving Access and Quality of Care are Indispensable Interventions for Reducing Maternal Mortality

Many of our countries in the Region of the Americas are going through an epidemiological transition, have different socioeconomic gradients, and display varying degrees of inequity. Therefore, we need to develop interventions for specific countries by using different approaches.

In the past, data on life expectancy, maternal and infant mortality, and causes of death were seen as sufficient for assessing population health status and determining public health priorities. As mortality rates have declined and life expectancy has increased, questions have arisen about the quality of life. The former indicators remain indispensable, as there are still major inequalities in mortality between countries and between groups within countries. Nevertheless, for a few countries in Latin America and the Caribbean, changes during the last 20 years have demonstrated the need for new indicators, namely disability-free life expectancy, healthy life expectancy, or active life expectancy. These indicators provide information on the functional state and vitality of the population as well as people's quality of life. These new indicators, which are appropriate for the epidemiological conditions of today, are not seen as a priority and are monitored in only a few Latin American and Caribbean countries, and this is another indication of the inequity among the countries of the region.

REFERENCES AND BIBLIOGRAPHY

Atrash H, Alexander S, Berg C. Maternal mortality in developed countries: Not just a concern of the past. *Obstetrics and Gynecology* 1995; 86(4) (ii).

Graham W, Brass W, Snow RW. Estimating maternal mortality: the sisterhood method. *Studies in Family Planning* 1989; 20:125–135.

Kennedy BP, Kawachi I, Prothrow-Stith D. Income distribution and mortality: cross-sectional ecological study of the Robin Hood index in the US. *BMJ* 1996; 312:1004–7.

Lozano R, Infante C, Schlaepfer L, Frenk J. *Desigualdad, pobreza y salud en Mexico.* Mexico, DF: Editora el Nacional; 1993.

Maine D, Rosenfield A. The safe motherhood initiative: why has it stalled? *American Journal of Public Health*, April 1999; 89(4).

Pinto da Cunha EMG. Raca; aspecto esquecido da iniquidad em saude no Brazil. In Barata, R.B. et al. (eds) Equidade e Saude. São Paulo, Brasil: Abrasco Huticet; 1997.

Robine JM, Romieu I, Cambois E. Health expectancy indicators. *Bulletin of the World Health Organization* 1999; 77(2).

UNICEF, WHO, UNFPA. Guidelines for Monitoring the Availability and Use of Obstetric Services; 1997.

Weaver J, Sprout R. Twenty-five years of economic development revisited. *World Development* 1993; 21(11).

WHO, UNICEF. The sisterhood method for estimating maternal mortality: guidance notes for potential users; 1998. (WHO/RHT/98.27).

Wilkinson RG. Socioeconomic determinants of health: health inequities: relative or absolute material standards? *BMJ* 1997; 314:591 (22 January).

World Health Organization. Maternal mortality ratios and rates: A tabulation of available information; 1991. (WHP/FHE/MSM/91.6)

HEALTH EQUITY IN RELATION TO SAFE DRINKING WATER SUPPLY

*Horst Otterstetter,[1,2] Luiz A. C. Galvão,[1] Vicente Witt, Peter Toft,[1]
Sergio Caporali,[1] Paulo C. Pinto,[1] Luiz C. R. Soares,[1] and Carlos Cuneo[1]*

INTRODUCTION

The United Nations Conference on Environment and Development, held in Rio de Janeiro, Brazil, in June 1992, issued a Declaration of Principles, asserting that "human beings are at the center of concern for sustainable development. They are entitled to a healthy and productive life in harmony with nature." The Conference's plan of action—Agenda 21—approaches environmental concerns and actions within a sustainable development process that focuses on the well-being of present and future generations. Section I of the Agenda, "Social and Economic Dimensions," emphasizes that the elimination of poverty and the protection and promotion of health are important elements of sustainable development (United Nations, 1992). Latin American and Caribbean countries took the position that, "There will not be sustainable development as long as almost half of the population continues to be in abject poverty." They further stated that, "Human development must

[1] Division of Environmental Protection and Development, Pan American Health Organization.

[2] The authors would like to acknowledge the contributions to this article by Division of Environmental Protection and Development's Country Advisors.

be the keystone of our strategy if it is to be ecologically viable. This, together with the rational use of natural resources, must be the central focus of our strategy. Every other concern must be subordinated to it." The Agenda also stresses that the achievement and maintenance of health for the Latin American and Caribbean population ". . . demands the integration of health concerns with those of the environment as part of the new model of sustainable development" (Latin American and Caribbean Commission on Development and Environment, 1990).

About 200 million poor live in Latin America and the Caribbean—in 1994, 38% of the total population was poor and 16% was indigent. Poor people in urban and rural areas by and large do not have safe drinking water supplies. Some carry water to their homes from stand pipes and consequently waste valuable work or study time and risk their health by carrying heavy loads and consuming unsafe water. Others purchase water from vendors at prices up to twenty times higher than that paid by people with piped water.

The implementation of Agenda 21 underscores the close and complex links between the environment and human health, as well as the need for decision-makers to have a broad understanding of the relationship between environmental risk and health outcome in order to control exposures and protect health, and concomitantly to contribute to the reduction of inequities. Unfortunately, even though the matter is of critical importance, it has been given limited attention so far, and there are few studies available on socioeconomic inequalities in access to safe water supply.

In addition to its marked interest in the issue of equity and health outcomes, the Pan American Health Organization (PAHO) also is concerned with equity in the various determinants of health, including the broad physical, social, and economic determinants of health. In many cases, the determinants of health are key to attaining equity in health.

Many determinants of health, as are determinants in other sectors, are linked directly or indirectly to poverty. Because the relationship between poverty and health, which has been known for centuries, is clearly evident today, PAHO is striving to identify and define inequalities and inequities in health status within and among countries. Through its various activities and programs, the Organization is trying to improve the knowledge about and understanding of this issue as a basis for diminishing health harms and risks, particularly for the more disadvantaged populations.

The relationship between health and the environment touches on an extremely broad range of issues. The ability to link health to environmental data, and to better understand how the physical, social, and economic environments affect health, continues to challenge health professionals. Nevertheless, this step is fundamental for controlling the adverse environmental effects on human health in general, and on the more disadvantaged groups, especially the poor, in particular. In order to establish these links, health and environment data must be analyzed as a way to estimate the health impact of environmental factors and set priorities for action according to the population's basic physical, social, and economic requirements (Associação Brasileira de Engenharia Sanitária e Ambiental, 1999; Associação Brasileira de pós-graduação em Saúde Pública, 1998; World Health Organization, 1996; World Health Organization, 1997).

The World Health Organization (WHO) has developed a six level cause-and-effect framework as a basis for analyzing how environmental risks generate health outcomes (World Health Organization, 1996). This framework, although still being tested, has provided valuable results that may help decision-makers and policy-makers understand these complex relationships and focus their actions on the health aspects of sustainable human development. This process should provide data to identify and better define where inequalities and inequities are concentrated and to determine which interventions are required to improve the situation.

In discussing the relationship among health, the environment, and sustainable development this chapter establishes a context for describing the basic situation that countries face in the new development processes. It also emphasizes the importance of water resources and the related inequalities that may affect the provision of safe drinking water supplies. This is a critical element among environmental determinants of health and an important expression of inequity, especially in relation to the health of the urban and rural poor. Further, this discussion demonstrates how water supply and sanitation measures affect populations, and how inequities in safe drinking water supplies can be demonstrated, specifically in relation to cost, coverage, and water quality. Finally, the chapter discusses the Environmental Health Framework for Decision-making, including the six lines of action designed to reduce inequities in relation to the provision of drinking water. It is expected that this methodology will be a useful mechanism for the identification, definition, prioritization, and implementation of actions to attain equity in health through environmental interventions.

HEALTH AND ENVIRONMENT IN HUMAN DEVELOPMENT

Inequalities and inequities in the provision of safe water have been expressed in many different ways and are considered explicitly in the broader global agenda on sustainable development. The Declaration of Principles issued in Rio de Janeiro, as expressed in Agenda 21, implies that development should meet the needs of people, their health, and their well-being, as well as provide a healthy environment in which people can attain their development, including health.

The basic human needs for a healthy environment are safe water, adequate food, and shelter, as well as the social and economic conditions whereby different people can live together with equity and peace—a desire of human beings over the ages. More recently, this aspiration has evolved into the concept of "human development" in the broadest sense, and is becoming a fundamental objective of more general development. Consequently, increasing awareness of the complex links between economic growth and environmental protection has become a major challenge in governments' efforts to achieve human-oriented sustainable development (Carey, 1999; United Nations, 1992; World Bank, 1999).

In the Region of the Americas, the subject of health and the environment in development has been discussed in several meetings of heads of state and, in particular, at the 1996 Pan American Conference on Health and Environment in Sustainable Human Development. Presently, governments and peoples are cognizant that they must reconfigure their development policies and programs to equitably meet growing human needs and to correct existing inequities, while at the same time maintaining an ecological balance and facing the pressing demand for constructing healthy social systems. It is important to keep in mind that insufficient development, which is generally a consequence of poverty—and poverty affects a very large portion of the population in developing countries in the Americas—can

be a major contributor to environmental deterioration; this, in turn, can result in poor health (Pan American Health Organization, 1998; Pfaff, 1999).

Currently in this Region there is an understanding of the fact that people's health cannot be promoted and protected by the health sector alone, or even primarily. As was shown during the Pan American Conference on Health and Environment in Sustainable Human Development in 1996, good health is the result of a series of actions by the whole of society, led by governments. Therefore, the establishment of partnerships that mobilize public and private sectors to act synergistically to address health goals is essential if significant progress is to be made. To fit within the framework of sustainable development, approaches to support health must shift from the traditional sectoral approach to a new, broader intersectoral effort. Intersectoral action is especially important when dealing with health and environment, because of the intrinsic links between the human and the natural environments (Pan American Health Organization, 1998; World Bank, 1999; Alleyne, 1998).

WATER RESOURCES AND QUALITY OF LIFE

Clean water is essential for life and for maintaining good health; it also is necessary for human activities, including those that enhance the quality of life. Except for some Caribbean islands, the Americas are endowed with a plentiful supply of surface water resources. About 13% of the world's continental waters are found in Latin America and the Caribbean. On a per capita basis, this Region is very rich in terms of water, compared with other continents, as shown in Figure 1, particularly since estimates of the amount of water needed for development indicate that countries with 1,000 m³ to 1,600 m³ per person per year may experience shortages in drought years, and that those with less than 1,000 m³ per person

FIGURE 1. Availability of water resources for human use, by region, 1970 and projections for 2000.

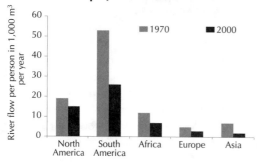

Source: Adapted from Reiff, 1989.

per year may see development curtailed (World Resources Institute, 1998).

Groundwater is a valuable source of drinking water supply, and most countries of the Region take care of the water supply needs of large populations using this resource. Although freshwater supplies in Latin America and the Caribbean vary significantly from country to country, few countries currently face problems nationwide. Nevertheless, several must deal with localized shortages of adequate drinking water sources, particularly in large metropolitan areas and in some smaller cities, where the poorer strata of the population are usually affected.

The need for water resources goes beyond quantity and must also consider quality. The capacity of these resources to provide water for human well-being is shrinking as a result of population growth, degradation from pollution and other environmental abuses, inefficiency, and waste. The poor can be further disadvantaged, as the areas they live in often receive effluents discharged by residents living upstream. Projections indicate that in the year 2000, the demand for water due to the increase of population alone will have doubled since 1980. The rate of increase is likely to grow further in future decades if appropriate policies are not implemented and appropriate actions are not taken.

The production of goods and services is necessary to meet the needs of ever-growing urban populations and improve the quality of life of the urban and rural poor. However, most of the uses of water contribute to degrade water quality, and this, in turn, affects human beings and other species that depend on this water for survival. In general, water quality must satisfy the requirements of society's many uses, but it is essential that drinking water meet public health requirements. Further, as pressure for different uses of water increases, the potential for conflicts also increases, with the risk that water quality for human consumption may fall by the wayside, thereby exacerbating existing inequalities. To avert severe conflicts relating to quantity and quality of drinking water, strong advocacy for new policies that give proper attention to water for human consumption is required. Presently, 2 billion people drink water that others would not even use to wash their cars, while another 1.2 billion people would dearly love to have such water (Otterstetter, 1996).

The quantity of water required by different users varies widely. On a global scale, needs for irrigation account for about two-thirds of all human water use: for example, it takes about 1,000 tons of water to grow 1 ton of grain, and some 2,000 tons to produce 1 ton of rice. However, these processes have associated water losses that may range from 50% to 80% (World Resources Institute, 1987), which means that there is room for improvement here. Reuse of municipal wastewater is another potential area of recovery for irrigation. In many cases, policies do not favor or give attention to the equitable distribution of scarce natural resources, such as the adequate assignment of water for drinking and other purposes. Frequently, the needs of the poor are ignored and, because of this, poor people often miss opportunities such as developing cottage industries or other activities that require water that could improve their economic status (World Bank, 1999).

In the Region of the Americas, it was estimated that 12% of the water consumed in 1995 was used for domestic purposes, while 26% was used for industrial purposes, with agriculture as the largest consumer (World Resources Institute, 1998).

DRINKING WATER SUPPLY AND HUMAN HEALTH

Water is an essential element in every aspect of human life: drinking, hygiene, cooking, and leisure. People are in contact with water all their lives and are exposed to whatever it contains. Water is also essential for other living organisms, including disease vectors.

Among all the uses of water and the needs of human beings, a safe drinking water supply is the most essential, although not sufficient in itself to attain and maintain good health. The association between safe drinking water and other sanitary measures to attain good health has been recognized for a long time. One example is the drop in diarrhea-gastroenteritis mortality rates in Costa Rica with the implementation of such measures (Figure 2). However, this knowledge is not always readily incorporated into water supply projects or other health and development projects. Figure 2 demonstrates the importance of water and sanitation to improve community health. Further, although the benefits are in many cases reaped by the better-off, the extension of coverage also usually benefits marginal areas to some extent (Alleyne, 1998).

An estimate of the impact of the exposure to poor water supply and poor sanitation on the risk of disease can be estimated on the basis of Disability Adjusted Life Years (DALYs). DALYs are the expression of the number of

FIGURE 2. Mortality rates from diarrhea and gastroenteritis versus time and percent of total population with improved water supply, Costa Rica.

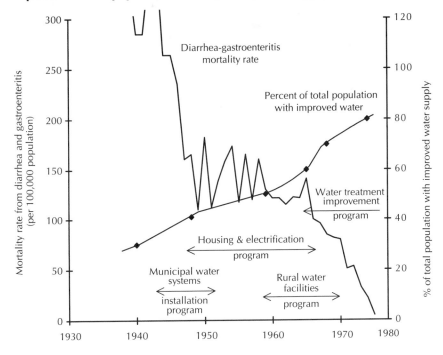

Source: Adapted from Reiff, 1981.

years of life lost (YLLs) added to a comparative adjusted measure of years living with disability (YLD). The YLD measurement adjustments are based on the severity and duration of the disease and age and sex of the individual (Murray, 1996).

For Latin America and the Caribbean, the DALYs of water- and sanitation-related risk factors is estimated at 5,183. This value means that water and sanitation are the most important environmental determinants of health—compared to determinants such as occupation and air pollution—and are more significant for this Region than malnutrition, which is the highest risk factor globally according to DALY calculation. Table 1 illustrates this data and reveals other related details. Unfortunately, there are no data available that specifically address low-income or poor populations (Murray, 1996).

Further illustrations of the association between the availability of water supply/sewerage/drainage and health indicators are shown in Figures 3 and 4. These figures are based on the results of a sanitary intervention in Baixa do Camarajipe, Salvador, Brazil, where a poor community received better sanitation from 1992–1998. As a result of these interventions, the level of diseases was reduced significantly (Borja, 1999).

The installation of water supply systems not only makes water available but also decreases the unit cost of water. This is particularly beneficial for the poor, who are subjected to paying high prices for limited quantities of water that is usually of questionable quality. Those

FIGURE 3. Decrease in the prevalence of diarrhea in children 0–5 years old due to improvements in sanitation in Baixa do Camarajipe, Salvador, Bahia, Brazil, 1993–1998.

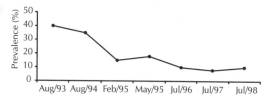

Source: Adapted from Borja, PC, Moraes, LRS, 1999.

who have no water or lack sufficient water are mostly poor, and for them the cost of water is higher than for the better-off, as shown in Figure 5. Consequently they use less water, and have lower levels of hygiene and a higher incidence and prevalence of several water-related diseases. There is no other way to break this vicious cycle than by improving access to adequate quantities of safe water through disinfected piped supply systems (Pan American

FIGURE 4. Decrease in the prevalence of helminthes infestation in children 7–14 years old due to improvements in sanitation in Baixa do Camarajipe, Salvador, Bahia, Brazil, 1994–1997.

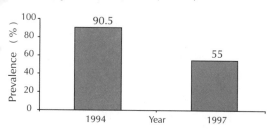

TABLE 1. Burden of diseases attributable to selected risk factors, Latin America and Caribbean, 1990.

Risk factor	Deaths (1,000)	% total deaths	YLLs[a] (1,000)	% total YLLs[a]	YLDs[b] (1,000)	% total YLDs[b]	DALY[c] (1,000)	% total DALY[c]
Poor water supply, sanitation, and personal and domestic hygiene	135.3	4.5	4,254	7.6	929	2.2	5,183	5.3
Malnutrition	135.0	4.5	4,540	8.1	520	1.2	5,059	5.1
Occupation	97.7	3.2	1,973	3.5	1,708	4.1	3,681	3.7
Air pollution	33.6	1.1	377	0.7	98	0.2	476	0.5

Source: Adapted from Murray, 1996. p.: 312–315.
[a] YLLs: Years of Life Lost; [b] YLDs: Years Lived with Disabilities; [c] DALYs: Disability-Adjusted Life Years.

FIGURE 5. Comparison of the cost of water between areas with and without water supply systems in selected countries of the Region.

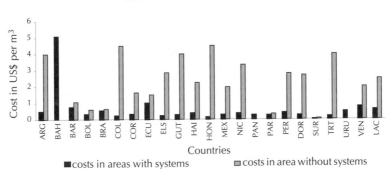

Health Organization, 1997). Evidence such as that shown in Figure 5 provides a strong argument that less than full coverage produces an unfair distribution of benefits and burdens; that is, inequities.

Even with the evidence available, governments often give a lower priority to investment projects for water supply and sanitation due to the cost. This may be due to a misconception of the role of water supply systems and sanitation, which, in addition to providing water for human consumption, are also an essential element of urban and industrial development. In the Region of the Americas only about 5% of the water supply produced is consumed directly for health-related purposes. Therefore, only about 5% of the cost of such investment should be considered a health-related cost. Furthermore, water systems are built with a projected life of 50 or 60 years; amortization of the investment should, therefore, be spread over this same period. By taking into account these two issues, investment in water supply becomes extremely cost beneficial in terms of improvements in health (Briscoe, 1996).

MEASURING INEQUITIES IN SAFE WATER SUPPLY

The main health inequities related to water supply deal with population coverage, quality, cost, and accessibility. Other factors, such as the geographic location of freshwater sources and the distance individuals must travel to gain access, accentuate existing inequalities.

To facilitate the analysis of the relationship between countries' economic level and the availability of water, information on countries in the Americas can be grouped on the basis of per capita GNP, according to the division adopted by PAHO. *Group I* includes the countries with the highest per capita GNP and *Group V*, the countries with the lowest per capita GNP (Table 2) (Pan American Health Organization, 1996; Pan American Health Organization, 1997; Pan American Health Organization, 1998).

In the Region of the Americas, 18% of the population has no access to water systems. In *Group V*, 43.8% of the population has no access and in *Group I*, 4.6% has no access. The ratio between the lowest and the highest GNP group of countries is 9.6, which means that the countries in *Group V* have 10 times more people without access to water than the countries in *Group I* (Figure 6) (Pan American Health Organization, 1997; Organización Panamericana de la Salud, 1998).

Inequalities also occur between rural and urban populations. In urban areas, 13.28% does not have access to water, while in rural areas, 40.58% has no access, indicating that the proportion of population without access to

TABLE 2. Country groups according to per capita GNP in 1996, population and population without access to water in 1998, and rate of population without water, Region of the Americas.

Groups	Per capita GNP, 1996	Population, 1998	Population without water, 1998	Rate of population without water (100 population)
GNP Group V	530.20	27,400,000	12,001,741	43.80
GNP Group IV	1,784.82	119,501,000	33,115,917	27.71
GNP Group III	3,497.49	307,332,000	73,073,052	23.78
GNP Group II	7,713.30	43,762,000	14,162,043	32.36*
GNP Group I	26,205.78	304,431,000	13,860,385	4.55
Region	11,986.29	802,426,000	146,213,138	18.22

Source: Pan American Health Organization, Special Program for Health Analysis.

* Group II included Argentina (Population, 36,123,000) and some small countries (Population, 7,639,000), as of PAHO basic data 1998. In Argentina, 65% of the population has access to water. Because the table uses average values for countries, the numbers for Argentina influence the rates of persons without access to water.

drinking water in rural areas is three times higher than in urban areas (Pan American Health Organization, 1997).

In rural areas, technical, educational, and socioeconomic limitations present additional challenges for securing high water quality. For example, supply systems in poorer, rural areas are less well maintained than are those in urban areas. In addition, the rural population has limited knowledge about the benefits of safe water, such as the need for adequate storage and disinfection.

Figure 7 presents the concentration curve and the concentration index for access to water in the Region of the Americas. To estimate these values, the groups of countries were ranked by GNP per capita, from the lowest to the highest. The concentration curve in Figure 7 suggests that in the Region of the Americas, 20% of the population that lives in countries with the highest GNP per capita have only 5% of their population without access to water. Conversely, 20% of the population of the region living in countries with the lowest GNP per capita have 30% of the population without access to water. A concentration index of –0.30 was estimated for this distribution (Kunst, 1994; Mackenbach, 1997; Pan American Health Organization, 1999).

Lack of access to basic sanitation services is directly associated with the incidence and prevalence of waterborne diseases and other health effects in the population. For example, there is a strong association between infant mortality and lack of access to drinking water, as shown in Figure 8. In areas where about 40% of the population has access to drinking water, infant mortality is about 50 per 1,000 live births, while in areas where 100% of the population has access to drinking water infant mortality is around 10 per 1,000 live births (Pan American Health Organization, 1999).

The above examples clearly indicate the need for strong policies for the provision of basic needs, especially drinking water supply, of marginalized populations in order to im-

FIGURE 6. Percent of population without access to drinking water in countries of Group V (lowest per capita GNP) and Group I (highest per capita GNP), Region of the Americas, 1995.

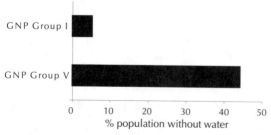

Source: Special Program on Health Analysis, Pan American Health Organization.

FIGURE 7. Distribution of the population without access to water in the Region of the Americas, 1997.

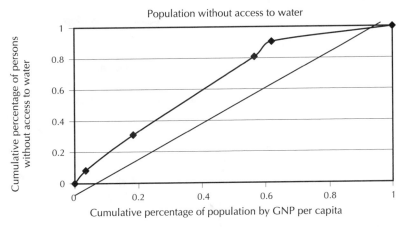

Source: Special Program on Health Analysis and Division of Environmental Protection and Development, Pan American Health Organization.

prove health and achieve equitable and sustainable human development, in accord with the spirit of the Rio Declaration and Agenda 21.

Under present economic conditions and trends, a country's ability to invest in water supply systems, improve coverage, and provide access to safe water depends largely on the population's ability to pay back the investments. Clean water is required for good health, but it also is a basic ingredient for urban development and for many industrial processes necessary to promote and sustain economic development. The development of water supply systems also must consider the benefit to other uses (externalities). Unfortunately, these

FIGURE 8. Trends in infant mortality rate (per 1,000 live births) and water access, Region of the Americas.

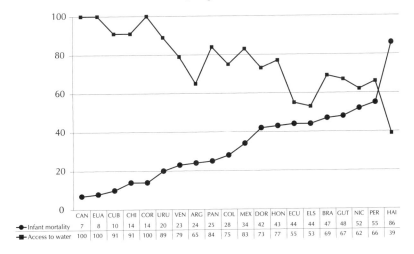

	CAN	EUA	CUB	CHI	COR	URU	VEN	ARG	PAN	COL	MEX	DOR	HON	ECU	ELS	BRA	GUT	NIC	PER	HAI
Infant mortality	7	8	10	14	14	20	23	24	25	28	34	42	43	44	44	47	48	52	55	86
Access to water	100	100	91	91	100	89	79	65	84	75	83	73	77	55	53	69	67	62	66	39

considerations are rarely given the weight they deserve, nor is cost-sharing generally incorporated into discussions (Rogers, 1997; World Health Organization, 1997).

ENVIRONMENTAL HEALTH FRAMEWORK FOR DECISION MAKING

The relationship between human health and the environment is complex, particularly since health/environment aspects are linked to several economic and social development issues. By and large, environmental data may be available in most countries, as may be data on the health situation. However, the ability to link health and environmental data to clarify the relationship between levels of exposure and health outcome is vital in attempting to control exposure and protect health. Decision-makers need this information in order to assess the implications of their decisions, compare the potential effect of different decisions, and prevent costly health and environmental damage (World Health Organization, 1996; World Health Organization, 1997; Brasil, 1999).

In order to tackle the problem, the World Health Organization, taking as a guide the model developed by the United Nations Development Program (UNDP) to monitor the progress of countries towards sustainable development, elaborated a framework for the analysis of various aspects of health/environment situations (World Health Organization, 1995).

WHO proposed a six-level, cause-effect framework as a way to facilitate the analysis of the environmental-health situation. The framework was designed to assist decision-makers and policy-makers in setting priorities and taking action, as well as to increase the focus on the health aspects of sustainable human development. It can facilitate the identification of inequalities and inequities as well as the development of actions to improve the situation (World Health Organization, 1995).

This cost-effect framework is known as DPSEEA, an acronym derived from its six action levels—driving force, pressure, state, exposure, effect, and action; it is a response to Chapter 40 of Agenda 21 (Information for Decision-making).

Driving force is the first and broadest of the framework's levels and refers to the general factors that motivate and drive environmental processes, such as population growth and economic development.

Driving forces generate human occupation or exploitation of the environment, resulting in *pressure* on the environment, which is the second level of the framework.

Continuing pressures alter the environment's original condition, leading to the third level of the framework—the *state* of the environment. An example of this level is the degree of balance between the natural components and the level of pollutants.

Environmental conditions and the presence of contaminants can result in environmental hazards for humans if they generate an *exposure*; this is the fourth level.

If an exposure exists, a health *effect* is expected to develop; this is the fifth causal-chain level. Health effects call for *action*, but the solution of the problem may require actions at all levels, or at certain levels of the causal-chain to attain the defined objective. Using the DPSEEA framework to orient these actions is critical if the health sector and other sectors are to achieve sustainable development. Figure 9 shows the dynamics of DPSEEA and the internal relations.

IDENTIFICATION OF PRIORITIES AND ACTIONS TO REDUCE INEQUALITIES

There are several actions that may be taken to reduce inequity in drinking water supply. Table 3 presents examples of lines of action that the health sector and other sectors may take at the different levels of the framework, emphasizing the practical application and use of the DPSEEA framework.

FIGURE 9. **Framework for decision making to mitigate inequities in water supply for human consumption and hygiene.**

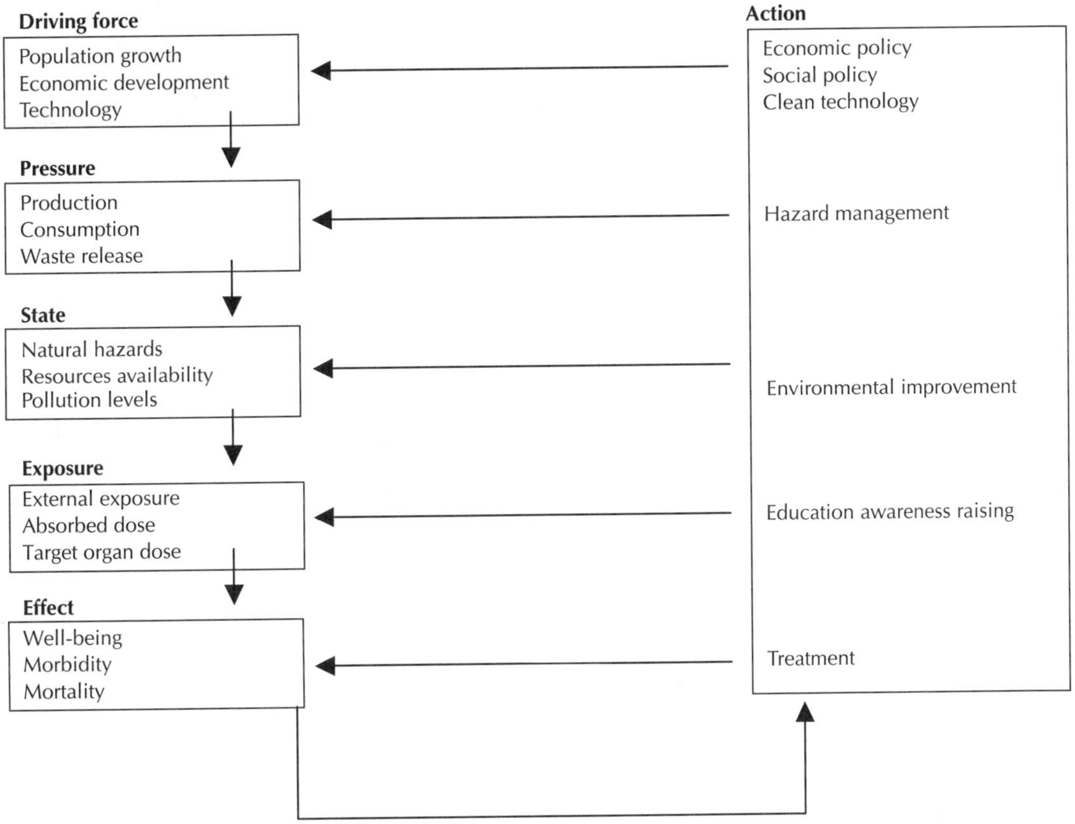

Source: Adapted from World Health Organization.

The examples included in the table take into account the importance of common lines of action to be explained later in the document. In applying DPSEEA to the health and environment area, it is important to consider at least five lines of action to change the situation:

- advocacy,
- regulations,
- monitoring,
- dissemination of technologies, and
- mobilization of resources.

LINES OF ACTION TO REDUCE INEQUITY

DPSEEA can generally use available information at the sector, institutional, and community levels to focus efforts and resources on priority interventions. The final actions to reduce the distributive gaps in drinking water supply that emerge from the application of DPSEEA should result in general lines of action that can be grouped into the five categories below.

TABLE 3. Actions to reduce inequity in safe water using the DPSEEA approach.

Cause/effect chain	Issues/examples	Health sector actions	Other sector actions
Driving force	• Urban and industrial development; • Housing and sanitation policies; • Poverty and social exclusion.	• Studies on implication of development policies in health; • Proactive role of the health sector in promoting sustainable development; • Advocacy before other sectors on adequate policies and regulation on water; • Promotion of the environmental primary attention strategy.	• Adopt health impact analysis in development projects and policies; • Include the health sector as a major contributor to national development plans; • Establish sound urban public health development policies.
Pressure on the environment	• Water supply for human and industrial consumption demand; • Housing and internal plumbing demand; • Sewerage and drainage systems demand.	• Promote use of appropriate and low cost technology for water supply; • Promoting healthy housing for the poor; • Promoting community participation; • Establishment of regulation for the control of pollution of the water bodies.	• Implement programs and projects for extension of coverage; • Implement system for the improvement of quality of water supply; • Implement regulation on population settlements and housing.
State of the environment	• Presence of pollutants in water bodies; • Pollution of drinking water; • Storage of water for human consumption in inadequate manner.	• Maintain environmental surveillance (monitoring and control) system; • Carry-out health education activities for hygiene and safe storage of water; • Advocate for projects on pollution control (wastewater treatment); • Monitoring water quality of the water supply systems.	• Maintain environmental surveillance system of water resources; • Implement pollution control projects (wastewater treatment).
Human *exposure*	• Consumption of contaminated drinking water; • Consumption of contaminated food.	• Implement community based demonstration projects; • Carry-out public education campaigns.	• Carry-out public education campaigns; • Implement community based demonstration projects.
Health *effects*	• Diseases and other effects that can be reduced by basic sanitation (diarrhea, hepatitis, parasitism, cholera, and low body weight and height development).	• Maintain epidemiological surveillance system of water-related diseases; • Improvement of health services.	• Cooperate with the health surveillance system; • Improve support of health services.

Monitoring Trends in Inequities in Water Supply

Existing inequities in safe water supply quantity and quality are relevant in explaining several health effects that are responsible for morbidity and mortality in the countries of the Region of the Americas. Existing mechanisms could be used to monitor inequities in water supply and could become powerful tools to identify deficiencies and to measure the health impact of improvements to the water supply. Therefore, it is important for countries to develop environmental and epidemiological surveillance systems.

The timely and updated data to maintain current the "Global Assessment of Drinking Water Supply and Sanitation Services 2000" database is expected to be a very important contribution to measure inequities and monitor changes in the Region.

Table 4 is an example of how DPSEEA can be used to establish indicators to measure inequities in water supply. A careful definition of the indicators to be used can assist decision-makers to focus their actions and scarce resources in areas where they can make a difference in the population's health.

Even though DPSEEA needs further evaluation and testing by international agencies and countries before being widely used, some pilot studies have already revealed that it can be a useful tool for supporting advocacy and dialogue among the sectors responsible for water supply and public health (Borja, 1999).

To further support the adoption of DPSEEA, PAHO has funded case studies, which have led to the establishment of a set of indicators to be used to analyze trends and generate critical information for actions.

At the international level, the database of the "Global Assessment of Drinking Water Supply and Sanitation Services 2000" is a major source of information. This initiative brings together critical information for analyzing water supply trends in the Region of the Americas, and most of it can be reassembled within the framework in order to make use of the data for both the environmental and the public health sectors. Efforts to obtain information on the situation of lower income population groups should take into account their concerns in the decision-making process.

National institutions also have their own databases and the same information that has been available for years for traditional analysis of trends can be integrated into the DPSEEA framework scheme, thus improving the planning and decision-making processes for the water supply sector.

TABLE 4. Use of the DPSEEA framework to establish indicators to measure inequities related to safe water.

Cause-effect chain level	Indicators
Driving forces	• Population Growth Index; • Percent of satisfied goals of national sanitation plan.
Pressure	• Percent of the population connected to a water supply system; • Median value of the consumed water in liters per inhabitant; • Median price of water expressed in percent of the median income.
State	• Percent of water samples with concentration higher than the national standard for *E. coli*; • Percent of samples without physical and chemical national standards.
Exposure	• Percent of population living in areas without any access to water supply.
Effects	• Incidence of acute diarrhea, intestinal parasitism, cholera, and low body weight and height development; • Number of health professionals trained for treatment of water-borne diseases.
Actions	• Percent of municipalities with environmental surveillance system; • Percent of municipalities with health education program.

Source: Adapted from Borja, 1999.

Strategies for Advocacy

The health sector alone cannot carry out all the functions required to secure a healthy human environment, but it can use advocacy to promote actions in other sectors that will help to reduce inequities in access to safe water supply. There are several examples where advocacy has influenced decisions in other sectors and has resulted in public health benefits. International agencies should play a strong role in providing evidence and international guidance to help country health authorities to effectively advocate for a healthy human environment. Other activities should include promoting intersectoral dialogue and actions; supporting country studies to generate data for advocacy; promoting the "Environmental Primary Attention Strategy;" and disseminating information.

Promotion to Strengthen Regulations

The health sector should fulfill its responsibility to develop and help implement regulations at the national level that contribute to reducing health inequities. The establishment of water quality standards and the maintenance of surveillance systems are some of the most important contributions that the health sector can make to the sustainable development of nations. The use of international guidelines for waste water and solid waste management and for drinking water quality, and the use of health impact assessments on plans, programs, and projects should assist countries in the implementation of national regulations.

Dissemination of Technologies

The lack of appropriate and economic technologies is frequently identified as a barrier for the development of a safe water supply. Experiences in several of the Region's countries have proven that investments in this area have clearly benefited health. The identifica-

tion, selection, and dissemination of information on technology can contribute at the same time both to reducing costs and to insuring selection of the most suitable technology.

Mobilization of Resources

The lack of financial resources is an important obstacle to the development of water supply in countries. The health sector can provide strong arguments to advocate for investment projects in this area, and also can develop studies to orient projects to maximize social and health benefits.

REFERENCES

Alleyne, G. A. O. Environmental management in Latin America and the Caribbean. Consultation Meeting on Environmental Management. Washington, DC: PAHO; 1998. http://www.paho.org/english/ops9813.htm

Alleyne, G. A. O. Environmental management in the twenty-first century. 26th Inter-American Congress of Sanitary and Environmental Engineering, Lima: PAHO; 1998. http://www.paho.org/english/ops9814.htm.

Associação Brasileira de Engenharia Sanitária e Ambiental; Brasil, Ministério da Saúde, Fundação Nacional de Saúde, Centro Nacional de Epidemiologia, Coordenação de Vigilância Ambiental; Organização Pan-Americana da Saúde: XX Congresso Brasileiro de Engenharia Sanitária e Ambiental: ABES/99: Oficina de Trabalho sobre indicadores de vigilância da qualidade da água para consumo humano. Relatório da oficina de trabalho. Brasília: 1999. http://www.fns.gov.br/cenepi/publicacoes.htm.

Associação Brasileira de pós-graduação em Saúde Pública — ABRASCO; Brasil, Ministério da Saúde — Fundação Nacional de Saúde — Centro Nacional de Epidemiologia — Coordenação de Vigilância Ambiental; Organização Pan-Americana da Saúde: Congresso Brasileiro de Epidemiologia — EPIRIO, Oficina de Trabalho sobre indicadores para a vigilância ambiental. Indicadores de Saúde e Ambiente. Informe Epidemiológico do SUS, Ano VII, No. 2 — Abr/Jun/98, p: 45-53. Brasília, Brasil, Resumos das Oficinas do EPIRIO 98. Brasil, 1998. http://www.abrasco.com.br/revistas/cienciaesaude/default.asp and http://www.fns.gov.br/cenepi/publicacoes.htm.

Borja PC, Moraes LRS. Relatório de projeto para a Organização Pan-Americana da Saúde: Uma contribuição para o estabelecimento de indicadores de

Saúde ambiental, com enfoque para a área de saneamento. Brasília, Brasil: OPAS; 1999.

Brasil, Ministério da Saúde, Fundação Nacional de Saúde, Centro Nacional de Epidemiologia, Vigilância Ambiental. Vigilância ambiental. Brasil; 1999. *http://www.fns.gov.br/cenepi/ambiental.htm.*

Briscoe, J. *Water as an economic good: the idea and what it means in practice.* The World Bank. A paper presented at the World Congress of the International Commission on Irrigation and Drainage. Cairo, September 1996. *http://www-esd.worldbank.org/rdv/training/icid16.htm.*

Carey G, Wolfensohn J. Creditors of the poor — yes, all of us: The Archbishop of Canterbury and the head of the World Bank speak out. *The Guardian* June 15, 1999. *http://www.guardianunlimited.co.uk/Archive/Article/0,4273,3875037,00.html#top.*

Kunst AE, Mackennbach JP. Measuring socioeconomic inequalities in health. WHO Regional Office for Europe, 1994. EUR/ICP/RPD 416. *http://saturn.who.ch/uhtbin/cgisirsi/CfwBWpU3CF/9457006/9*

Latin American and Caribbean Commission on Development and Environment. Our Own Agenda. IADB/UNDP, New York, 1990.

Mackenbach JP, Kunst A. Measuring the magnitudes of socio-economic inequalities in health: an overview of available measures illustrated with examples from Europe. *Soc. Sci. Med.* 1997; 44 (6). *http://oxford.elsevier.com/cgi-bin/JAO/A-/pass?a=SSMAO&j=SSM &c= abstract&B =+aff&b=JRNL+V00044N006+ 96000731 #aff*

Murray CJL. Rethinking DALYs. In Murray CJL, Lopez AD. (eds.) *The Global Burden of Diseases.* Global Burden of Disease and Injury Series, vol. I. Cambridge: Harvard University Press; 1996.

Organización Panamericana de la Salud. *Informe Anual del Director, 1995: En busca de la equidad.* Washington, DC: PAHO; 1996. (Documento Oficial No. 277).

Organización Panamericana de la Salud. Situación de Salud en las Américas: Indicadores Básicos 1998. Washington, DC: OPS; 1998. (OPS/HDP/HDA/98.01).

Otterstetter Horst. Agua: en búsqueda de la equidad. Conferencia regional sobre reforma y moderación de los servicios de agua potable y saneamiento para México, Centroamérica, Haití y la República Dominicana. Honduras, 1996.

Pan American Health Organization. *Health in the Americas, 1998 edition.* Vol. I. Washington, DC: PAHO; 1998. (Scientific Publication No. 569).

Pan American Health Organization. *Annual Report of the Director, 1998: Information for Health.* Washington, DC: PAHO; 1999. (Official Document No. 293). *http://www.paho.org/english/Annrep-98/report-index.htm#top*

Pan American Health Organization. Mid-decade evaluation of water supply and sanitation in Latin America and the Caribbean. Washington, DC: PAHO; 1997.

Pfaff ASP, Stavins RN. Readings in the field of natural resource and environmental economics. The World Bank Web page, June 22, 1999. *http://www.worldbank.org/nipr/readings/readings.pdf.*

Reiff F.M. The impact of agriculture and industrial development on Latin America and the Caribbean. American Society of Civil Engineers meeting, USA, 1989.

Rogers P, Bhatia R, Huber A. Water as a social and economic good: how to put the principle into practice. The World Bank Group, November 1997. *http://www-esd.worldbank.org/rdv/training/watroger.htm.*

The World Bank Group. World Bank's World development indicators: Indicators-on-the-web, Water — Quality — Pollution. *http://www-esd.worldbank.org/eei/; http://wbln0018.worldbank.org/environment/EEI.nsf/all/Environmental+Indicators?OpenDocument.*

The World Bank Group. Competitiveness indicators. *http://wbln0018.worldbank.org/psd/compete.nsf/e24271d1df909fb38525650c005d9097/ab417cfa708544f58525650c005d9367?OpenDocument*

The World Bank Group. Expanding the measure of wealth: indicators of environmentally sustainable development. *http://wbln0018.worldbank.org/environment/EEI.nsf/3dc00e2e4624023585256713005a1d4a/aa228cb86afc7ec18525671c00570418?OpenDocument.*

United Nations Organization, Secretariat of the United Nations Commission on Sustainable Development. United Nations Conference on Environment and Development (UNCED); 1992. (Agenda 21.) *http://www.un.org/esa/sustdev/agenda21.htm.*

United Nations Organization, Secretariat of the United Nations Commission on Sustainable Development. United Nations Conference on Environment and Development (UNCED); 1992. (Agenda 21, Chapter 40, Issues: Indicators.) *http://www.un.org/esa/sustdev/isd.htm*

World Health Organization. Sustainable Development and Healthy Environments Cluster, Department for Protection of the Human Environment (PHE), Water, Sanitation and Health (WSH). Water, Sanitation and Health at WHO-HQ. *http://www.who.int/water_sanitation_health/Watsanhealth/WSH_brief.html.*

World Health Organization. WHO report Health and Environment in Sustainable Development: Five Years after the Earth Summit. Geneva: WHO; 1997. *http://www.who.int/environmental_information/Information_resources/htmdocs/execsum.htm*

World Health Organization. Linkage Methods for Environment and Health Analysis. General Guidelines. A Report of the Health and Environment Analysis for Decision-making (HEADLAMP) project, edited by Briggs D, Corvalán C, Nurminen M. Geneva: WHO; 1996. (WHO/EHG/95.26).

World Health Organization. Linkage Methods for Environment and Health Analysis. Technical Guidelines. A Report of the Health and Environment Analysis for Decision-making (HEADLAMP) project, edited by Corvalán C, Nurminen M, Pastides H. Geneva: WHO; 1997. (WHO/EHG/97.11, v + 153 pages).

World Health Organization. Focus in environmental health indicators. *GEENET Newsletter* 1995; 6. *http://www.who.int/peh/geenet/archive/geeupdt6.html*.

World Health Organization. The Global Burden of Disease project (GBD). Global Burden of Disease and Injury Series. *The Executive Summary of the Global Burden of Disease and Injury Series. http://www.hsph.harvard.edu/organizations/bdu/gbdsum/gbdsum5.pdf*.

World Resources Institute. *World Resources 1998–99: A Guide to the Global Environment—Environmental Changes and Human Health*. New York: Oxford University Press; 1998. *http://www.igc.org/wri/wr-98-99/index.html*.

ACCESS TO AND FINANCING OF HEALTH CARE: WAYS TO MEASURE INEQUITIES AND MECHANISMS TO REDUCE THEM

Daniel López Acuña,[1] César Gattini,[1] Matilde Pinto,[1] and Bernt Andersson[1]

INTRODUCTION

Health systems and services primarily aim at contributing to the promotion and restoration of health status, as well as engaging in disease prevention and palliation for the whole population. However, health needs vary from person to person, which implies that there is a need for different types of interventions, both within and outside the health sector. Health care delivery then becomes an organized answer to various health needs through differential health care interventions.

Conditions in the health services and the population's health needs are subject to multiple factors related to the socioeconomic context. Socioeconomic development is linked not only to better health (lower health care needs), but also to higher financing and availability of health service resources, and to better access to health care.

The measurement and analysis of inequities in access to and financing of health care, including determinant factors influencing supply and demand of health care, are essential for monitoring the implementation of mechanisms aimed at reducing those inequities.

[1]Division of Health Systems and Services Development, Pan American Health Organization.

The objectives of health reform in the Americas include improving equity in service delivery, improving efficiency in management, and increasing the effectiveness of actions—all of which are necessary to meet the health needs of the population. Within this context, equitable access to effective health services is one of the guiding principles of Latin American and Caribbean health sector reform.

The First Summit of the Americas, held in Miami, Florida, in 1994, established a plan of action to guide national health sector reforms, including a specific initiative (Initiative 17) for achieving equitable access to basic health services. The central objective of the Latin American and Caribbean Health Sector Reform Initiative, which was launched in 1997, is to provide regional support to the promotion of equitable access to basic quality services in the Region of the Americas.

As part of the initiative, PAHO has developed a methodology to monitor and evaluate health sector reforms in Latin America and the Caribbean. This methodology entails the preparation of profiles on the countries' health systems and services as a way to establish the current health status baseline, in order to measure the impact of reforms. Additionally, PAHO is developing an instrument to monitor the effects of reforms on equity in access and utilization of health services.

This chapter examines the assessment of inequities in access to and financing of health care and the ways to measure and analyze inequities; it also presents a proposal to reduce inequities in both access to and financing of health care.

ASSESSING EQUITY IN ACCESS TO AND FINANCING OF HEALTH CARE

Assessing inequalities in access to and financing of health care involves the measurement and analysis of inequities, beginning with a measurement of *disparities*, or inequalities. An analysis of *inequities* involves applying a value-laden judgement to variations beyond certain range that are considered unfair or unjust, under normative criteria, and/or the lack of correspondence between the patterns of distributions in health care resources and health care needs.

The concept of inequity involves the notions of vertical and horizontal equity in health care. This, in turn, involves acknowledging that different health needs must be treated differently (vertical equity) and that people with equal needs ought to be treated equally (horizontal equity), regardless of ability to pay or any other socioeconomic characteristic.

The analysis of equity-related variations—i.e., those disparities or inequalities that have a connotation of inequity—must consider the health system framework in which the variations occur. This supports the analysis of inequities within real settings. The choice of ways to measure and analytical methods will depend on the measurement purposes, information availability, and the background of the real setting where variations are being analyzed.

Differential health situations, especially avoidable morbidity and mortality, are determined by multiple factors, with health care being just one of them. There are multiple models supported by statistical associations and causal relationships which give accounts of the relative weight of the factors that affect differential health status of the population; these factors include socioeconomic context, physical and geographical environment, lifestyles and health behaviors, biological and demographic conditions, and *health care*. Most of these factors are also determinants for differential access and use of health care.

Multiple perspectives and measures are then needed to address this issue comprehensively. We need to combine them all within a coherent conceptual and methodological framework. Such an approach to address the problem of inequities in access and financing should take into account that:

- From the supply side, several institutional factors lead to the availability of health services to different target populations.
- From the demand side, several factors facilitate access to services according to need, regardless of ability to pay.
- The utilization of health services represents effective access to health care, assumed to be the result of the interaction between supply and demand factors.

Barriers to health care—such as geographical, economic, cultural, and economic obstacles—need to be taken into account, but there also are other factors that influence access to and utilization of health services. The whole set of factors that influence the use of services and the satisfaction of health care needs within an iterative circle of *need→demand→use*, makes the analysis of equitable cross-sectional distributions of health care more complex.

Most of these factors are interrelated and play a role in a process whereby health needs are sometimes expressed as health demands, some of which result in the utilization of personal and public health care, provided it is available and accessible. Therefore, access to health care cannot be assessed through a single, distinct measurement of a discrete event, as is the case for most health outcome measures.

In the pursuit of equity, the challenge for health systems is to attain a balance between the health needs of the population and the availability of organized resources supporting the provision of services to satisfy those needs.

Equity in health care is, therefore, pursued through three components:

1) a *needs-based role for health services*, which seeks to deliver services according to need, irrespective of sex, age, ability to pay, ethnicity, culture, or place of residence.
2) a constant pursuit of *allocative efficiency*, which searches for the best possible combination and distribution of health care benefits by setting priorities in the allocation of resources according to the epidemiological profile and cost-effectiveness of the interventions (health value for money); and
3) the search for *productive (or technical) efficiency*, to ensure that the available resources can support the best possible provision of care, adapted to the populations' needs and demands.

Social, economic, and health disparities between different areas and population groups influence the delivery of health care. Underprivileged areas tend to have a higher burden of disease, lower availability of resources, lower financing and access, shortages of health care personnel, lower prestige, and a limited capacity to solve health events that require more complex, technological levels of care; this is described as the inverse health care law (Hart, 1971).

Multiple factors related to socioeconomic development and incentives to providers (public or private) influence the supply of services. These factors include the financing of the system, the level of investment in the sector, the training of qualified personnel for the health services, and the allocation and efficient use of existing resources.

Measurement and analysis of inequities in access to and financing of health care is both a problem- and policy-oriented issue, and it can become a tool in the search for solutions to inequities, such as removal of barriers to access, specific investment in health care, and the search for improvement of efficiency and effectiveness of health services.

MEASURING AND ANALYZING INEQUITIES IN ACCESS TO AND FINANCING OF HEALTH CARE

Important preconditions for the adequate assessment and analysis include the clarification of the purpose of measurement and the availability of appropriate information, including characteristics of the health system to be analyzed.

The availability of information should ideally cover a wide range of data from both the supply and demand sides, including the population, health status, health services (including access, use, and financing of health care) as well as the determinants for variations of all these factors.

Two main sources of information are used in measuring access to health care. The first is household surveys and other surveys that gather information on health needs and demands, patterns of utilization of services, and problems faced by the individuals in accessing health services. The second source is the use of routine statistics gathered within the health system, including data from health information systems, such as morbidity and mortality statistics.

The measurement of variations in access to health care must take into account the issues mentioned in the preceding paragraph and must establish meaningful parameters for comparison within a country and among countries. This involves selecting variables and categories of analysis such as geographic areas, income quintiles, educational level, race, ethnicity, type of insurance coverage, or institutional affiliation, provided that the information from either surveys or health care providers' statistics can be broken down by those categories.

To obtain a comprehensive picture of health care inequities that focus on access and financing, one must compare measurements of different dimensions of the process: availability of resources, access to health care, and utilization. The analysis is greatly enriched when variations in the distribution of these resources are compared to differential patterns of health care needs.

The coexistence of public and private services in most countries, involving different health care networks that provide services to different populations sharing a common geographical area, implies the need to integrate information on those different providers and target populations. It also implies the requirement of different information sources, integrated under common criteria and standards.

Availability of Health Care Resources

Availability of resources (at the geographical and institutional level) can be measured using a variety of indicators that are generally produced by all countries. Indicators such as those listed below must be stratified by various population groups in order to make distributional comparisons.

- Health expenditure and sources of financing:
  - public health expenditure per capita,
  - household contribution to sector financing, and
  - financing in personal care and public health.
- Availability of physical and human resources:
  - doctors or nurses per 10,000 inhabitants and
  - hospital beds per 10,000 inhabitants.

Administrative data is normally available for geographical areas, but often only for public resources. Information is not so readily available for the private sector. Geographical areas can be homogeneous and give a good picture of social or economic inequities, if the area is populated by one ethnic group or by people in the same income group. However, an area often can encompass a mixture of ethnicity and socioeconomic groups, or it has no registered information. Data are often not available for different income groups, ethnic groups, or professions; one may have to rely on special studies or surveys to obtain this data. One strategy is to find ways to disaggregate routine data to smaller geographical areas.

As an example of data supporting the comparison of resources per population, Figure 1 shows the availability of hospital beds in Latin American and Caribbean countries.

Measuring Access to Health Care

Access to health care often is measured only by geographic and economic barriers, including insurance coverage. Cultural and social factors also present access barriers to care, however. Measurement of the effect of cultural and social factors in access involves a sociological approach to the pathways to health care, which is not necessarily reflected in geographic and economic measures.

Geographic Access to Health Care

The assessment of geographic access is commonly approached by measuring the time individuals must take to cover the distance between their households and the health services, at least primary health care facilities. This indicator is subject to limitations of interpretation in relation to the concept of access. However, this indicator could become a useful proxy for geographical access in countries or areas where limitations of health care geographical coverage are important, due to the existence of rural and dispersed populations or the lack of health care centers.

Beyond simple geographical distance to health services, variations in access measured by this indicator depend on such factors as availability of proper transportation or roads and the existence of natural obstacles (rivers or mountains). This also means that geo-

FIGURE 1. Hospital beds per 1,000 inhabitants, in Latin American
and Caribbean countries, trends 1964 to 1996.

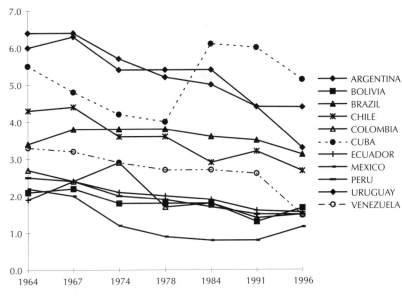

Source: 1964–1991: *Health Conditions in the Americas,* PAHO, 1998.

graphic access can change over time, as roads
or transportation conditions may improve.

Financial Factors Related to Health Care Access

Degree of Social Protection in Health

One of the variables indicating inequities in
health care is the affiliation of various groups
with social insurance for health. Salaried workers and their dependent families who work in
the formal economic sector normally have the
obligation to make financial contributions in
order to be covered by public health insurance
(or some scheme of social security) or private
insurance. In Latin America, it is estimated that
about 55% of the population is covered by a
social insurance scheme for health care.

Low-income workers in the informal sector are for the most part not affiliated with any

public or private insurance. Their only protection for health comes from direct out-of-
pocket payments for health care to private or
public facilities or from subsidized care in
public sector facilities provided through governmental policy. Health coverage for this seg-
ment of the population is generally less comprehensive than that available for people who
work in the formal sector.

Although the situation may vary somewhat
from country to country, generally those excluded from health insurance schemes are
found among the poor, the elderly, women and
children, indigenous groups, workers in the
informal sector, the unemployed, and the rural population. Therefore, it may be helpful to
analyze data according to categories that high-
light these socioeconomic groups, and to examine differences between the population
covered and not covered by the different types
of schemes.

Financial Burden Associated with Access to Health Services

The financial burden includes the cost of direct out-of-pocket payments, fees, and drugs; from the household perspective, there also is a cost for travel and lost income, which adds to a total expense for health that is higher than the flow of funds that go to the health system. No routine data is normally available, so in this case also, one must rely on studies and surveys.

The significant household participation in health sector financing is an aspect of financing inequities. Household expenditure includes contributions to any health insurance as well as out-of-pocket expenditures. Information on National Health Accounts for eight Latin American and Caribbean countries estimated that household participation in health sector financing fell within a range from 31% in Bolivia to 79% in the Dominican Republic (Table 1). These results contrast with those in more developed countries: in the United Kingdom, Spain, France, the Netherlands, Italy, and Denmark, for example, household expenditures represent between 8.4% and 30.0% (Wagstaff and Doorslaer, 1999).

This financing pattern is inequitable, since expenditures for health services represent a greater proportion of the income for poor families than for wealthier ones. By relating patterns of private health expenditure to the

TABLE 1. Household participation in health sector financing, selected countries in Latin America and the Caribbean, 1999.

Country	Household participation in health sector financing (%)
Bolivia	31
Dominican Republic	79
Ecuador	33
El Salvador	53
Guatemala	55
Mexico	64
Nicaragua	32
Peru	37

Source: LAC/HSR Initiative, PAHO/USAID. National Health Accounts: Eight country studies in Latin America and the Caribbean; 1999.

level of per capita income in countries of the Region, an inverse relationship can be observed (with some exceptions) between the percentage of private health expenditure and total health expenditure as it relates to per capita GDP.

UTILIZATION OF HEALTH CARE

The utilization of health services is influenced by health needs, gender, socioeconomic status, ethnicity, and cultural factors. An additional challenge for the measurement of access is to take stock of the differential patterns of utilization of various services, i.e., ambulatory care, hospital care, emergency medical services, immunization, rehabilitation services, prenatal care, etc. Such an effort calls for the development of a core set of indicators of access to health care that is clustered by types of services and sensitive enough to allow for monitoring and evaluation of trends and changes in this area.

Some of the indicators that can be used to measure the utilization of health services are:

• outpatient visits per capita of target population,
• utilization of hospital beds per 100 of target population,
• coverage of prenatal care,
• coverage of professional childbirth delivery, and
• coverage of immunizations.

Table 2 shows the number of medical consultations per inhabitant in Peru's departments, grouped according to poverty index.

The availability of data is the major shortcoming for measuring inequities in access to health care at different levels within a country. To measure access, utilization indicators such as the number of outpatient medical visits per person or hospital admissions per person are commonly used. Data on utilization assume that data collected by health centers refers mainly to the target population within

TABLE 2. Selected indicators of health and health care in departments grouped in quintiles ranked by poverty, Peru, 1997.

Indicator	Q1	Q2	Q3	Q4	Q5
Population data					
Population (millions)	3.9	3.7	3.7	4.8	8.3
Poverty (%)	65.9	57.8	52.4	40.8	28.5
Life expectancy (years)	62.8	65.8	66.4	70.4	76.6
Utilization indicators					
Doctors/1,000 population	3.3	5.0	6.2	8.9	18.6
Hospital beds/1,000 population	1.1	1.5	1.3	1.9	2.4
Medical consultations/inhabitant	0.6	0.8	1.0	1.3	1.9
Hospital admissions/1,000 population	17.0	26.6	32.9	48.7	63.4

Source: Elaborated from MINSAL Perú - OPS (1998). Situación de salud de Perú. Indicadores básicos 1997.

a defined catchment area (which has to be verified). However, this assumption is limited by the cross-boundary flow of patients.

These indicators are based on routine data; however, national information systems on utilization of services seldom include socioeconomic data or data on race, ethnicity, culture, or religion of users (patients visiting hospitals or health centers), and do not include data of potential users within the target population who do not have access.

Survey data can then be used to characterize a given area according to categories of variables such as the population's socioeconomic status, race, ethnicity, culture, or religion, as well as by coverage by social insurance for health. Data from surveys is complementary to routine data; both could be used jointly when exploring the characteristics of those using and not using health services within a catchment area, or comparing usage between different areas.

PAHO's Division of Health Systems and Services Development (HSP) is currently working on an instrument for monitoring equitable access to basic health services that takes into account the issues raised in this paper. It will be field-tested and made available to Member Countries as soon as it is revised. The instrument includes indicators of health outcomes, utilization of services, and availability and accessibility to resources, as well as structural indicators.

Countries in Latin America and the Caribbean have different levels of socioeconomic development, ill-health status, and availability and use of health care, as well as different patterns of geographical variations in these variables. However, it is possible to find similar patterns across countries, as described in the inverse care law.

This can be illustrated with some selected data from indicators of socioeconomic circumstances, health, and health care, based on data already available for geographical areas within those countries.

Figure 2, based on data from Peru's 25 departments, ranked by poverty, demonstrates the relationship between the population's socioeconomic development (represented here by the reduction of poverty in geographic areas) and infant mortality rate (a proxy for health needs), as well as access to and use of services (represented by the ratio of medical consultations and hospital admissions per population). Improvements in health and health care occur in areas with greater socioeconomic development, while more deprived areas have the lowest levels of health and health care.

The distributional pattern tends to be systematic, supporting the inverse care law. One risks bias in these comparisons if causality is assumed, but research on causality is hindered by the circularity of health care needs, demand, and use. The context of multiple and

FIGURE 2. Differential pattern of health (infant mortality rate) and
access/use of services (medical consultations and hospital admissions)
in departments ranked by poverty, Peru, 1997.

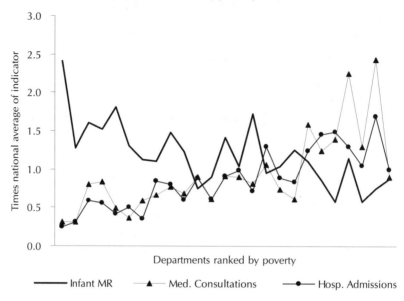

Source: MINSAL-OPS Perú. Indicadores básicos situación de salud 1997.

interrelated macro determinants of health makes it difficult to search for attributable impact of health services. There are only a limited number of studies and most of these are cross-sectional, which makes it difficult to infer causal explanations. From the knowledge in the current literature, one can make educated guesses to analyze variations in health care and those factors which are assumed to be determinant on access to and financing of health care services.

The analytical description of differential use of services according to differential needs for health care may be illustrated in data such as those used in Figure 3—this figure shows differences in the ratio of public and private hospital admissions per 100 population in groups of communes in Chile in 1992. These groups are ranked by potential years of life lost (PYLL) from 0 to 64 years of age, taken as a proxy for health care needs. Quintile 1 is the group of

FIGURE 3. Public and private hospital admissions per 100 population, by residence, in groups of communes ranked by potential years of life lost (0 to 64 years),[a] Chile, 1992.

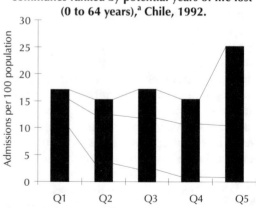

Source: Gattini, C., 1996.
[a]Ratio PYLL 0–64 years per 1,000 population, used as proxy for health care needs.

communes with the highest PYLL and admissions have been measured by commune of residence.

In this example, the group of communes with the lowest health care needs (Q5) has the highest ratio of hospital admissions per 100 population, mainly by getting access to private hospitals and specialties in public hospitals. The other quintiles (Q1 to Q4) have similar ratios of hospital admissions. Admissions to general medicine increase clearly towards quintiles with higher PYLL, compensating for the progressive reduction of admissions to public hospital specialties and private hospitals.

A similar pattern could be seen when communes are ranked by socioeconomic development, due to the relationship between socioeconomic factors and differential health care needs (if represented by PYLL). These data reinforce the importance of locating general hospitals in poorer and rural areas, as well as locating general medicine services within more complex hospitals, where needs are higher.

REDUCING INEQUITIES IN ACCESS TO AND FINANCING OF HEALTH CARE

The identification of mechanisms to reduce these inequities calls for a systemic examination to address the underlying causes of avoidable limitations to access in certain population groups. Some of these problems can be effectively solved within the boundaries of the health care system, while others will require the participation of other institutions in the social sector at the government level, particularly regarding the role of public sector financing.

Inequities in access and financing are due to factors that may reinforce each other's impact. In general terms, health care financing options are not neutral regarding equity. Progressive financing is the most equitable method of financing health services. It can be achieved through direct public funding (with revenue from taxes), through social health insurance schemes that cover the entire population, or through a combination of these two. Direct user fees constitute the most regressive and inequitable method of health care financing (Dahlgren, 2000). Experience indicates that high user fees pose significant economic barriers to access to health services.

A country's health care financing strategy should be designed by selecting the combination of mechanisms that simultaneously promote financial sustainability and provide equity. Studies of patterns of health care services utilization indicate that among those with perceived illness, "financial problems" are an important reason for not seeking care when needed. These financial problems are in part explained by financing strategies that require patients to make financial contributions, as well as by the lack of adequate insurance available to the population. The areas of health system organization and health care financing strategies can provide mechanisms to reduce disparities that are inequitable.

A systemic strategy to increase access to services should simultaneously implement mechanisms to increase the availability of providers (with an emphasis on the areas which present shortages of provision) and increase expressed demand to satisfy health needs. Increasing demand should be accomplished by lowering financial barriers, expanding social protection, and improving users' accurate perception of illness.

Proposals for the expansion of social protection in health must address factors both external and internal to the health sector. External factors exist largely outside the health system, and include the society's overall socioeconomic status, level and distribution of poverty, state inefficiency in both collecting and distributing resources, and model of development. Internal factors are closely linked to the health system. Obviously, the health sector is not powerless in responding to external factors, nor can it necessarily modify internal factors at will. A primary challenge is to determine at which level of dialogue issues should be addressed when cooperating with external actors.

Among internal factors, there are structural barriers that are due to the system's degree of fragmentation. Usually, health care is provided by the following four subsectors within the health system.

a. The *public sector*, usually provided by the central government, is based on overall taxation and is free to all users.
b. *Social security*, usually provided by specialized institutions, is based on payments by formal-sector workers and employers (although sometimes voluntary membership is possible); it is free but restricted to members (and occasionally their families).
c. The *private sector*, usually based on a pay-per-service system or funded by insurance schemes where a periodic fee or premium is collected, offers services restricted to paying patrons.
d. The *voluntary sector*, usually provided by nongovernmental organizations (NGOs) or community services (including either insurance or services, or both), is mainly oriented to the poorer population. This sector compensates for the exclusion or lack of coverage by the more "conventional" sectors mentioned above. For this reason, this sector is also known as *alternative* or *complementary* to the conventional sectors.

REDUCING BARRIERS TO EFFECTIVE ACCESS

Structural Barriers

There are three levels of intervention to reduce structural barriers:

1. Improving access within the mandate of each subsector (an internal question).
2. Strengthening the sector's leadership to effectively reach agreement among the first three subsectors (the conventional subsectors) to unite or at least cooperate to avoid duplicating actions and coverage.
3. The growth of the voluntary subsector can be understood because it is not clear how far

the conventional subsectors can respond and provide access to the entire population in an effective and efficient manner while respecting cultural values. The question, then, is not how to avoid the voluntary subsector (where it is justified), but rather how to ensure that it provides a reasonable level of health to the population it affects. Furthermore, this subsector is unlikely to be able to afford all levels of attention. Thus, the extension of social protection in health will have to include the articulation of the conventional and voluntary sectors for *services* that are beyond those the latter can reasonably provide (i.e. spinal cord surgery). By the same token, the insurance component of the voluntary sector will need to be linked to the national (public and/or private) insurance system for the purposes of reinsurance and coverage of catastrophic situations that might ruin the voluntary system.

Financial Barriers and Financing Inequities

A review of the health care financing components in a given country, along with an analysis of information on utilization patterns by specific groups (the poor, the elderly, the unemployed, indigenous peoples, etc.), will provide an initial assessment of inequities in health financing as well as financial barriers to access to care. The concept of inequity in financing is related to what proportion of household income each income group must devote to health care. Mechanisms should be implemented to reduce the share of financing among low-income households, whether through health insurance premiums (private or public), payment of fees to formal providers (in the public or private sector), payment to informal providers, or self-medication.

In the course of identifying mechanisms to reduce inequities in health financing, the role of public financing in the redistribution of resources will have to be given significant attention. Public financing can be targeted to reduce low-income families' financial contributions when those contributions reduce access or increase inequities.

To attain the goal of guaranteeing access regardless of a family's ability to pay, a combination of traditional mechanisms and complementary financing mechanisms should be employed. Traditional mechanisms include (a) public financing (through taxes), (b) user fees, (c) private health insurance, and (d) national health insurance. Complementary mechanisms are those aimed at compensating vulnerable groups for the effects of financial barriers, which lower their demand for health care.

Among traditional financing mechanisms, user fees have proven to reduce access to health care, while access to private (for-profit) health insurance has no potential to reduce inequity, since ability to enroll is determined by ability to pay. Complementary mechanisms are subsidies to the provision of care to vulnerable groups for reasons such as poverty, medical condition, or age. They can be implemented by publicly financing a social insurance scheme targeted to a specific beneficiary population. By definition, subsidies are to be paid using public resources, which requires that providers who normally charge for their services be financially compensated for providing services to the beneficiary populations. This is a crucial point in the analysis of providers' behavior, and it directly affects the possibility of increasing availability of services.

REDUCING CULTURAL AND ETHNIC BARRIERS

Studies of utilization patterns for health services often face difficulties regarding differing perceptions of illness and attention to preventive care among different population groups. Studies of health needs show that low-income groups express demand below their relative need. Thus, some mechanism is needed to narrow the gap between need and actual demand.

This issue is closely related to the organization of health systems, insofar as systems should be responsive to users' knowledge and perception of health problems. In some countries, responsiveness will include an ability to deal with language barriers. The creation of a population of educated consumers requires a core strategy of health education.

INCREASING AVAILABILITY OF HEALTH CARE SERVICES

Availability of services is closely related to availability of financial resources. A set of incentives that promote health care provision to population groups who have lower access will encourage providers to increase supply to areas or population groups with reduced access. Provider payment mechanisms can be successfully used to influence the availability and makeup of services to be offered. These mechanisms may include differential payment to foster provision in specific geographical areas as well as among priority populations.

Better utilization of available and limited resources can effectively increase the availability of health care. A more productive combination of inputs involved in the health care delivery process can help achieve technical efficiency, so that more services can be offered using the same amount of resources. By the same token, improvements in health service management can translate into successful increases in health care availability.

Another strategy would involve revising the health care model to make it more responsive to the epidemiological profile of the population to be served, as well as following criteria of cost-effectiveness in defining the package of care to be provided.

Because there are many factors that can cause inequities in access to care, multiple dimensions of the problem must be considered in attempting to reduce gaps in access to care. It also is important to identify the institutional factors that hinder or support equitable access policies in real settings. All this requires an integrated information system that covers multiple dimensions, uses several sources, and is supported by functional networks.

Both efficiency and equity can be fostered through a system of health care delivery (whether public, private, or mixed) that is organized in a multilevel basis. As long as referral from one level to another is based on need, such a system can provide appropriate access, not only to primary health care, but also to more complex levels of care.

CONCLUSION

In order to ensure access to health care according to need—and irrespective of age, sex, ability to pay, ethnicity, or cultural aspects—this discussion proposed a comprehensive framework for equity in access to and financing of health care. The first component addresses methods to measure and analyze avoidable disparities, which is followed by a proposal of policies and mechanisms to reduce inequities in access to and financing of health care. In order to document inequities, the chapter emphasizes the need to use a set of complementary mechanisms, multiple indicators, and information sources on socioeconomic circumstances, health needs, allocation of resources, and the use of health care.

However, in addition to documenting inequities, it is important to implement and evaluate mechanisms aimed at reducing disparities in access to health services and financing of health care.

Although there are some good indicators of equity, health sector information systems rarely register information about ethnicity, income, occupancy, or any other socioeconomic characteristics on a routine basis. Data unavailability is the major shortcoming for measuring inequities in access to health care.

There are basically two sources of information: 1) vital statistics and data from health sector activity registries and 2) population surveys on access to services. From a techni-

cal standpoint, it would be ideal to combine vital statistics and health registry data with the data obtained through access surveys.

The most widely used way to measure equitable access involves administering surveys to a representative sample of the population. However, the process is expensive, involves the participation of large numbers of personnel, and requires very complex statistical analysis. Although some of these difficulties may diminish somewhat as surveys are repeated, significant financial resources will always need to be outlaid for their execution.

On the other hand, routine statistics already provide information from different sources, but data usually do not address differential access between subgroups in the population. A strategy for overcoming this limitation involves collecting data that is as disaggregated as possible for small area levels.

Several mechanisms are proposed to improve equity in health care. These mechanisms pursue a dual purpose: creating a needs-based delivery of services irrespective of ability to pay, and constantly pursuing efficiency in the allocation of resources (value for money).

Taking into account the need to reduce barriers to effective access and improve availability of health services, some of the measures that can be implemented for ensuring and improving equitable access to health services are the following:

- increasing the availability of services, particularly to underserved areas;
- relying on public funds to finance the utilization of services by the most vulnerable groups (defined by socioeconomic or epidemiological criteria);
- reducing cultural and/or ethnic barriers to health care access and providing care in an intercultural context;
- diminishing the segmentation of health services networks (public and private) so they can cover different groups of the population;
- improving the integration of the health care delivery networks, in order to facilitate access irrespective of insurance coverage;

- expanding social protection in health by incorporating segments of the population currently excluded from social health insurance; and
- reducing the financial burden for accessing services, with an emphasis on the poor.

Monitoring equitable access to basic health services is crucial, as is documenting the impact of different policies and strategies in terms of effective reduction of disparities in access to health care. All of this should be part and parcel of PAHO's priority lines of action in the area of health systems and services.

REFERENCES

Dahlgren G. Efficient equity-oriented strategies for health. *Bulletin of the World Health Organization* 2000;78 (1).

Gattini C. Needs and equity in health care. The case of the National System of Health Services in Chile. HSRU, LSHTM, U. of London; 1996. (Draft report).

Hart J. T. (1971) 'The inverse care law.' *Lancet* 1: (696) 405–412.

Perú, Ministerio de Salud, Organización Panamericana de la Salud. *Situación de salud en el Perú. Indicadores básicos 1997.* MINSAL/OPS; 1998.

Pan American Health Organization. *Health in the Americas, 1998 edition.* Washington, DC: PAHO; 1998.

Pan American Health Organization, Division of Health and Human Development, Public Policy and Health Program. Health Expenditure Database. Washington, DC: PAHO; 1998. (Latest revision, September 1998).

Pan American Health Organization, Division of Health Systems and Services Development. Clearinghouse on Health Sector Reform in Latin America and the Caribbean. Washington, DC: PAHO; 1999.

Pan American Health Organization. Managing and Financing Health to Reduce the Impact of Poverty in the Caribbean: Implementing Decentralization and Financing Strategies while Protecting the Poor. Washington, DC: PAHO; 1999.

Wagstaff A, Van Doorslaer E. (1993) Equity in the finance and delivery of health care: Concepts and definitions. In Van Doorslaer E, Wagstaff A, Franz R. (eds.) *Equity in the finance and delivery of health care. An international perspective.* Commission of the European Communities HSR Series No. 8. Oxford: Oxford University Press; 1993.

Wagstaff A, Van Doorslaer E. Equity in the finance of health care: some international comparisons. *Journal of Health Economics* 1999; May.

PART 3

MAKING HEALTH EQUITY
WORK AT THE COUNTRY LEVEL

EQUITY AND HEALTH: A CARIBBEAN PERSPECTIVE

Richard A. Van West-Charles[1]

Any discussion of equity and health must take place within a context that focuses on creating an environment that enables human beings to enjoy long, healthy, and creative lives. Hence, the discussion of equity and health must revolve around human development, which denotes the process of widening people's choices and improving their level of well-being and capacity for self-empowerment. In its conceptual framework, UNDP has identified the following life conditions as critical to well-being:

- a long and healthy life,
- education,
- a decent standard of living,
- political freedom,
- guaranteed human rights, and
- self-respect.

When one considers these life conditions, they all seem so subjective that their interpretation varies from individual to individual, population to population, and community to community, based on one's culture, belief system, resources, etc. Notwithstanding this difficulty, one can make a quick identification of populations that exist in poverty. These populations are unable to contribute to their own individual growth and to the growth and development of their respective communities.

When discussing the topic of equity and health, many are immediately drawn to focus on poverty. In many instances, however, this focus is motivated by benevolence rather than development, and presents limitations in terms of social benefit. It permits solutions to be passive and more conscience-relieving than dynamic and demonstrative that the existence of poverty is a deterrent to the creation of global well-being and development. Poverty concentrates on deprivation of three essential elements: longevity; knowledge; and a decent standard of living.

- Deprivation of longevity relates to survival and vulnerability to death at an early age, specifically, life expectancy under 40 years.
- Deprivation of knowledge relates to being excluded from the world of reading and communication.
- Deprivation of a decent standard of living comprises three variables: percentage of people with access to health services, of people with access to safe water, and of malnourished children under the age of 5 years.

These deprivations define vulnerable populations who require specific investments so they can have the opportunity to survive and participate in the development process. Hence, in terms of our discussion for action on health and equity, these vulnerable populations must be identified, not because of a

---

[1] PAHO/WHO Representative, Bahamas.

moral imperative but rather for a development imperative.

Having addressed the need to protect these vulnerable populations, let us turn our attention to the rest of the population in terms of equity and health in the developmental context. The barriers to an individual's or a population's quest for well-being are related to the determinants of health, including economic status, communication resources, the environment, the health/medical system, knowledge/access to information, and gender. In each of these areas, barriers to the attainment of well-being can be defined, identified, and studied epidemiologically. For example, Epi-data, which points to an increasing incidence and prevalence of asthma, can point to factors that require intervention and investment at different levels.

CURATIVE

As the balance of health determinants shifts, disease processes are manifested in relation to people's exposure to physical, chemical, or biological agents. Hence, the health system's curative component is central to the re-establishment of well-being, and the organization of the health system becomes a pivotal consideration. But the medical model construct cannot be considered sufficient. This paradigm of the health system, of which the curative component is a part, must reflect an active understanding of the role of the determinants in the manifestation of disease and attainment of well-being.

HEALTH FACILITIES/TECHNOLOGY

The relevance of health facilities and technology to health equity must be considered within the context of the global, national, and regional environments, and within these environments, in terms of the private and public sectors as well as the nongovernmental and community-based organizations.

Participatory planning with the involvement of all sectors can lead to equitable development and can support environments that promote health and well-being, resulting in priority programs reflective of epidemiological analyses and research.

TECHNOLOGY

An important aspect of the health care delivery system in relation to health equity is the availability of technology. The use of technology must be assessed based on its contribution to the well-being of the entire population. Because the availability of technology is dependent on very limited resources, its equitable contribution to health depends on analyzing who is in greater need. Access issues are relevant not only to the use of public resources to achieve health and well-being, but also to the use of private sector resources, a sector that is not always held to the same equity standard as the public sector. There should be no difference in terms of the basic permissible standards for the public sector, private sector, and nongovernmental organizations. For example, the availability of mammography for women, be it in the public or private sector, must meet standards for the equitable application of the technology.

Public resources must be used first to benefit the vulnerable groups of a society—not in a manner which will deter the generation of greater wealth, but with the intent of contributing to empowerment in a way that balances with other components of the society. This obviously cannot be done solely by the sector that is responsible for the contribution of health to development, but rather must be accomplished in dynamic partnership with other sectors.

The indices that will assist in the development of a formula for the maximization of resources and its greatest empowerment are:

• public expenditure ratio—percentage of national income that goes into public expenditure;

- social allocation ratio—percentage of public expenditure earmarked for social services;
- the social priority ratio—percentage of social expenditure devoted to human priority concerns;
- the human expenditure ratio—percentage of national income devoted to human priority concerns.

Clearly, depending on the philosophical forces in a society, the analysis of these ratios can be performed in different ways, such as focusing on the public and/or private sectors, thereby permitting different responses, all of which may be considered equitable. But the use of these ratios in any analytical approach would require further analysis as to whether the socially allocated resources are inappropriately aimed at curative health and therefore neglect to invest in broader determinants of well-being.

FINANCING

Discussions of financing structures for attaining health and well-being must include an understanding of global, regional, and national financing frameworks and the values that inform them.

Two components comprise the financing of well-being and health. The first is based on consumer choices and expenditures on activities related to determinants, e.g. binge dieting versus nutritious choices or water rates versus fashion. This component depends on a high level of literacy which, when combined with information, creates greater opportunity for consumers to choose healthy behaviors. The second component is related to how the curative component of the system is financed. If we recognize that resources are required to support a system that involves technology, and if quality assurance is to be maintained equitably, then technology must be accessed by all of society, and the system must have guidelines to ensure that standards do not vary according to individuals' ability to pay, e.g. access to mammography for early detection of breast cancer.

ACCESS

Access is not determined solely by physical access, but rather can be considered to have three components:

(a) *physical access*—a facility is provided where services are offered.
(b) *clinical access*—the provider is available and delivers a high standard of service in accordance with established norms. Clinical access also depends on the setting. For example, the operational norms and standards for an ICU vary with the mechanisms for financing in the private and public sector, or, outsourcing of staff in critical units can undermine or compromise continuity of care that is urgently needed. This does not mean that outsourcing is irrelevant, but rather that within the reform agenda, guidelines need to be developed to ensure that the financing agenda is in sync with the developmental objectives of equity and health.
(c) *therapeutic access*—many patients, especially the elderly, are unable to purchase the pharmaceutical agents prescribed, and as a result, the full attainment of the health equity objective is inhibited.

In many circumstances for a significant percentage of the population (a) and (b) become operative and (c) is very difficult to meet whether in part or whole.

EFFICIENCY/EFFECTIVENESS AND EQUITY

Many who have addressed the topic of efficiency and effectiveness seem to conclude that it is difficult for efficiency/effectiveness and equity to complement each other. But achieving equity is dependent on the effective use of resources and technical efficiency, and any equity proposal should explain how the resources are to be distributed, and how effective and efficient that distribution has been in the past or can be. In the context of development, the equitable use of resources must meet certain criteria, one of which is sustainability. The search for equity, then, must be approached through multiple steps for any given issue that affects human health. For example, immunization contributes to both individual and societal development. Likewise, when dealing with vulnerable populations, resources must target basic determinants that affect individuals' health and that of the population at large. Hence, resource allocations should consider that society cannot develop if large sections live in poverty or vulnerable conditions. Also, resources must be invested within a structure that maintains human capital. In the end, the resources must be well targeted if efficiency and effectiveness are to contribute to equitable development.

Análise de Eqüidade – Saúde: Brasil

Jacobo Finkelman[1]

MARCOS REFERENCIAIS

A *reforma sanitária* brasileira tem como marco de debate a 8ª Conferência Nacional de Saúde realizada em 1986,[2] propondo ampla reestruturação financeira, organizacional e institucional do setor público de saúde, com três objetivos principais: a) transferir a responsabilidade da prestação da assistência à saúde do governo da União para os governos locais; b) consolidar o financiamento e a provisão de serviços públicos de saúde, orientando-os para a eqüidade, a universalidade e a integralidade da atenção; e c) facilitar a participação efetiva da comunidade no planejamento e controle do sistema de saúde.

A Constituição Federal de 1988 dedicou à saúde uma seção no capítulo da Seguridade Social. O texto constitucional configura a saúde como um direito de todos e um dever do Estado, sob a garantia de políticas econômicas e sociais dirigidas tanto para a redução dos riscos de doenças e outros agravos à saúde, quanto para o acesso universal e igualitário às ações e serviços de promoção, proteção e recuperação da saúde, num *sistema único de saúde — SUS*, de caráter público, federativo, descentralizado, gratuito, participativo e de atenção integral.

Esse marco constitucional gerou as chamadas *Leis Orgânicas da Saúde* (8.080/90 e 8.142/90), o Decreto 99.438/90 e as Normas Operacionais Básicas — NOBs, editadas em 1991, 1993 e 1996. A Lei 8.080/90 regulamenta o SUS, que é responsável, ainda que sem exclusividade, pela concretização dos princípios constitucionais do direito à saúde. O SUS agrega todos os serviços públicos (de níveis federal, estadual e municipal) e os serviços privados, quando credenciados por contrato ou convênio. As NOBs, por sua vez, a partir da avaliação dos estágios de implementação do SUS, voltam-se mais direta e imediatamente para a definição das estratégias aplicáveis em cada momento de construção do Sistema e dos respectivos processos para a sua operacionalização.

As mudanças institucionais propostas sinalizam para a implementação de medidas estruturais, compreendendo:[3] a) um processo de mudança cultural e de afirmação da cidadania, em que a saúde é valor permanente e qualificador da vida; b) a consolidação de um sistema público nacional, em que as três esferas de governo atuem de modo complementar e harmônico, dispondo dos instrumentos de po-

---

[1] Representante da OPAS no Brasil.
[2] Brasil, Ministério da Saúde. *Anais da 8ª Conferência Nacional de Saúde, 17–21 de março 1986*. Brasília: Centro de Documentação do Ministério da Saúde; 1987.

[3] Brasil, Ministério da Saúde. *Informe sobre a reforma do setor saúde no Brasil*. Documento elaborado para a reunião especial sobre a reforma setorial do setor saúde, promovida pela OPAS, BID e Banco Mundial. Brasília, setembro de 1995.

der necessários; c) a organização e regulamentação de um sistema assistencial privado, com objetivos específicos solidários aos preceitos de assistência universal, integral e eqüitativa; d) o funcionamento competitivo dos subsistemas público e privado, estimulador da qualificação com redução de gastos; e) a adoção de modelos técnico-operacionais inovadores, que visem a atenção integral, individual e coletiva; f) a implantação de um sistema de acompanhamento, controle e avaliação; g) a introdução de práticas de gestão descentralizada e desconcentradora, que evitem processos cumulativos ineficazes e injustos.

O sistema brasileiro de serviços de saúde está formado por uma rede complexa de provedores e financiadores, que abarca os segmentos público e privado. O segmento público engloba os provedores públicos dos três níveis de governo, que no nível federal são o Ministério da Saúde (gestor nacional do SUS), os hospitais universitários do Ministério da Educação e os serviços próprios das Forças Armadas. Os níveis estadual e municipal compreendem a rede de estabelecimentos próprios das respectivas instâncias. Esse sistema cobre cerca de 75% da população. Os planos e seguros privados de assistência à saúde estão agrupados em quatro grandes categorias: (a) *medicina de grupo*, representando 47% do mercado de serviços privados; (b) *cooperativas médicas*, com 25% do mercado; (c) *planos de saúde de empresas*, com 20% do mercado; e (d) *seguro-saúde*, com 8% do mercado. A cobertura dos planos e seguros privados atinge 20% da população brasileira.

Os marcos referenciais apresentados pressupõem clara intencionalidade política e institucional, no sentido de dotar o país de condições para promover a eqüidade possível no campo da saúde. No entanto, a intencionalidade doutrinária tem encontrado dificuldades de contextualização no quadro de limitações econômico-fiscais existentes, gerando certo grau de frustração de expectativas, apesar de significativos avanços quantitativos alcançados na cobertura dos serviços.

ABORDAGENS SOBRE A EQÜIDADE

Uma forte característica da sociedade brasileira é a presença de altos níveis de desigualdade socioeconômica. Um recente estudo produzido pelo BID concentrou-se essencialmente no papel da educação como gerador de desequilíbrios de renda. Não deve ser esquecido, porém, que uma das faces mais cruéis dessa disparidade encontra-se precisamente na área da saúde, embora os estudos realizados na área não tenham dado a devida importância a essa questão.[4]

As medidas de desequilíbrio da eqüidade em saúde podem compreender diferentes categorias de análise, entre elas: a) a percepção do estado de saúde; b) a demanda por serviços; c) os gastos com saúde; d) os perfis de saúde; e) a prestação de serviços; f) o financiamento da saúde. Essas categorias devem ser analisadas comparativamente segundo condições sociais, econômicas e geográficas.

Há premente necessidade de esforços para desenvolver metodologias de análise e monitoramento das questões de eqüidade na área da saúde, de forma a construir indicadores específicos e estudar suas correlações com a disponibilidade de renda das pessoas, em diferentes situações geográficas e socioeconômicas.

O tópico seguinte apresenta uma apreciação linear dos indicadores disponíveis, entre os de maior impacto, comparando-se áreas geográficas que reconhecidamente se situam em escalas diferentes de desenvolvimento socioeconômico.

ANÁLISE DE INDICADORES SELECIONADOS

Condições de vida

Análises baseadas na aplicação do Índice de Desenvolvimento Humano — IDH, utilizado

---

[4] Campino ACC et al. *Equity in Health in LAC – Brazil.* 1998. (Documento fotocopiado).

pelo Programa das Nações Unidas para o Desenvolvimento — PNUD, situam o Brasil entre os países de médio desenvolvimento humano em 1997[5] (índice de 0,739), ocupando o 79º lugar no *ranking* mundial.

- A comparação do IDH entre as grandes regiões e os estados pode ser analisada em estudo divulgado em 1998 pelo PNUD-IPEA, com base em dados de 1991, que mostra disparidades significativas (IDH-M).[6] O Brasil e todas suas regiões apresentam-se no estrato de médio desenvolvimento, com expressivas variações regionais, desde o Nordeste (0,517) até a Região Sul (0,777). Em relação às unidades da federação, apenas o Distrito Federal situou-se no estrato superior de desenvolvimento humano (0,806), seguido dos estados de São Paulo, Rio Grande do Sul, Santa Catarina e Rio de Janeiro, com índices superiores a 0,780. Quatro estados apresentam valores abaixo de 0,500, situando-se, portanto, no estrato inferior de desenvolvimento humano: Maranhão, Piauí, Alagoas e Paraíba. Próximos ao limite inferior do estrato intermediário, situam-se os estados do Rio Grande do Norte, Sergipe, Bahia e Ceará, com índices inferiores a 0,540. Ressalte-se que todos os oito estados com os menores índices estão localizados na Região Nordeste.
- A renda média dos 10% mais ricos é cerca de 30 vezes superior à dos 40% mais pobres, enquanto que em países com grau de desenvolvimento comparável ao do Brasil é apenas 10 vezes maior.[7] Os 50% mais pobres tiveram, entre 1960–1990, sua participação na renda nacional reduzida de 18% para 12%, enquanto a renda dos 20% mais ricos elevou-se, no mesmo período, de 54% para 65%.
- Em 1997, a razão de renda entre os 20% de renda superior e os 20% de renda inferior nas areas urbanas do país foi de 18,9 na média nacional, variando de 26,4 no Maranhão a 9,7 em Roraima.[8]
- O perfil da concentração de renda no país pode ser apreciado na análise do coeficiente de GINI para 1997. Para o Brasil o coeficiente se situa em 0,588, variando de 0,556 no Sul a 0,606 no Centro-Oeste.[9]
- Em 1990, o salário médio das mulheres correspondia a 63% do recebido pelos homens. As disparidades étnicas evidenciam-se nos menores rendimentos percebidos por pretos e pardos, contingente que representa 45% da população do país e cujo salário médio correspondeu, em 1990, a 68% dos recebidos pelos brancos.[7]
- Na média brasileira, os pobres (indivíduos com renda familiar per capita de até meio salário mínimo) constituíam, em 1997, 28,4% da população, 45,1% dos quais residentes na região Nordeste. Nas médias regionais, o Nordeste apresentava-se com 52,2% de pobres na composição de sua população total, seguindo-se o Norte, com 34,5%; o Centro-Oeste, com 22,6%; o Sudeste, com 16,0%; e o Sul, com 19,1%. Entre os estados, a proporção de pobres variou de 9,9% em São Paulo a 64,2% no Maranhão.[10]
- Em 1995, 10% das crianças de 7 a 14 anos não freqüentavam a escola, proporção que atingia 15% na região Nordeste.[11]
- A taxa de alfabetização da população com 15 ou mais anos de idade era de 85,3% em 1997, com equivalente distribuição por se-

[5] Programa das Nações Unidas para o Desenvolvimento (PNUD). *Relatório do Desenvolvimento Humano 1999*. Lisboa: Trinova Editora; 1999.

[6] IPEA, PNUD, IBGE, FJP-MG. Atlas do desenvolvimento humano no Brasil. CD-ROM, 1998.

[7] Programa das Nações Unidas para o Desenvolvimento (PNUD), Instituto de Pesquisa Econômica Aplicada (IPEA). Disparidades sócio-econômicas. Em: *Relatório sobre o desenvolvimento humano no Brasil*. Brasília: 1996.

[8] Fundação IBGE. Razão de renda. Em: *Rede Interagencial de Informações para a Saúde (RIPSA). Indicadores e dados básicos Brasil, 1998*. Brasília: IBGE; 1999.

[9] Fundação IBGE. Pesquisa Nacional de Amostra por Domicílios (PNAD). 1997.

[10] Fundação IBGE. Taxa de pobreza. Em: *Rede Interagencial de Informações para a Saúde (RIPSA). Indicadores e dados básicos Brasil, 1998*. Brasília: IBGE; 1999.

[11] Fundação IBGE. Diretoria de pesquisas. Em: *Pesquisa Nacional de Amostra por Domicílios (PNAD). Síntese de indicadores 1995*. Rio de Janeiro: IBGE; 1996.

xos. A Região Sul apresentava a taxa mais elevada do país (91,7%) e a Nordeste a mais baixa (70,6%), destacando-se o estado do Maranhão com a taxa de 64,2%, a menor do país.[12]

- Em 1997, 34,9% da população com 10 ou mais anos de idade tinham menos de 4 anos de estudo, proporção que variava de 53,4% na Região Nordeste a 25,8% na Região Sul. Os estados do Maranhão e Piauí apresentavam os menores níveis de escolaridade (59,7% e 59,0%, respectivamente), enquanto no Distrito Federal apenas 19,0% da população nesse grupo etário tinha menos de quatro anos de estudo.[13]
- Da população entre 10 e 14 anos de idade em 1997, 16,9% estavam ocupadas (trabalho infantil), percentual que se eleva a 24,0% na Região Nordeste, atingindo 37,7% no estado do Maranhão. As menores taxas corresponderam à Região Sudeste (10,8%) e ao Estado do Rio de Janeiro (5,1%).[14]
- Dados de 1990 relacionam o trabalho infanto-juvenil com a renda familiar,[7] mostrando que a taxa de atividade das crianças de 10–14 anos era de 23% entre as famílias pobres, e de apenas 4,5% entre aquelas com rendimento familiar per capita acima de dois salários mínimos.
- A expectativa de vida ao nascer era de 67,8 anos em 1997, sendo de 64,1 para homens e de 71,7 para mulheres, mostrando uma sobrevida de 7,6 anos a favor do sexo feminino. Comparando regiões e estados, observa-se que a expectativa mais baixa encontra-se no Nordeste (64,8 anos), sendo a menor no estado de Alagoas (59,3).[15] A Região Sul apresenta a melhor expectativa de

vida (70,3 anos), mais elevada no Rio Grande do Sul (71,0).

- A taxa de fecundidade total foi calculada, para 1997, em 2,4 filhos por mulher ao longo de todo o período reprodutivo, com variações de 3,3 na Região Norte (máximo de 3,6 no Acre) a 2,1 no Sudeste (mínimo de 2,0 no Estado do Rio de Janeiro).
- A proporção da população com 65 e mais anos de idade alcançou 5,4% na média nacional em 1996, com valores extremos nas regiões Norte (3,3%, com 2,4% em Roraima) e no Sudeste (5,8%, com 6,7% no Rio de Janeiro).

Situação de saúde

- A mortalidade infantil no Brasil é estimada em 37,4 por mil nascidos vivos para 1997, variando de 58,3 na Região Nordeste a 24,0 na Região Sul. Os valores extremos entre os estados são observados em Alagoas (74,1) e no Rio Grande do Sul (19,7).[16]
- No grupo de menores de 5 anos, 5,7% dos óbitos informados no Brasil em 1997 foram devidos à doença diarreica aguda. Esse percentual é mais elevado na Região Nordeste (9,3%) e mais baixo nas regiões Sudeste (3,2%) e Sul (3,8%).[17]
- A prevalência de déficit ponderal em menores de 5 anos de idade foi estimada para 1996 em 5,7% na média nacional, variando de 8,3% na Região Nordeste e de 7,7% na Região Norte, até 2,0% na Região Sul.[18]
- Na Região Nordeste concentraram-se 98,4% dos casos de cólera registrados no país em 1997, expressando condições de vida parti-

[12] Fundação IBGE. Taxa de alfabetização. Em: *Rede Interagencial de Informações para a Saúde (RIPSA). Indicadores e dados básicos Brasil, 1998*. Brasília: IBGE; 1999.

[13] Fundação IBGE. Níveis de escolaridade. Em: *Rede Interagencial de Informações para a Saúde (RIPSA). Indicadores e dados básicos Brasil, 1998*. Brasília: IBGE; 1999.

[14] Fundação IBGE. Trabalho infantil. Em: *Rede Interagencial de Informações para a Saúde (RIPSA). Indicadores e dados básicos Brasil, 1998*. Brasília: IBGE; 1999.

[15] Fundação IBGE. Esperança de vida ao nascer. Em: *Rede Interagencial de Informações para a Saúde (RIPSA). Indicadores e dados básicos Brasil, 1998*. Brasília: IBGE; 1999.

[16] Fundação IBGE. Estimativas de mortalidade infantil. Em: *Rede Interagencial de Informações para a Saúde (RIPSA). Indicadores e dados básicos Brasil, 1998*. Brasília: IBGE; 1999.

[17] Brasil, Ministério da Saúde, CENEPI. Mortalidade proporcional por doença diarreica aguda em menores de 5 anos. Em: *Rede Interagencial de Informações para a Saúde (RIPSA). Indicadores e dados básicos Brasil, 1998*. Brasília: Ministério da Saúde, CENEPI; 1999.

[18] BENFAM. Pesquisa nacional de demografia e saúde. Em: *Rede Interagencial de Informações para a Saúde (RIPSA). Indicadores e dados básicos Brasil, 1998*. Brasília: BENFAM; 1999.

cularmente favoráveis à transmissão da doença na região.[19]

- A prevalência de hanseníase em 1997 situou-se, na média nacional, na taxa de 5,4 por 10 mil habitantes, variando de 15,0 na Região Norte a 2,7 na Região Sul. O estado com maior taxa foi Mato Grosso, na região Centro Oeste (19,0). Seguem-se os do Amazonas (17,4) e Roraima (16,2). No Maranhão, na Região Nordeste, a taxa foi de 14,5%. Todos os estados da Região Norte apresentam taxas superiores a 12,0. Os estados do Rio Grande do Sul e Santa Catarina apresentam taxas inferiores a 1,0, considerando-se a doença já eliminada como problema de saúde pública.

- A incidência de câncer cérvico-uterino, que é passível de prevenção na atenção básica à saúde, apresenta elevadas taxas nas regiões Norte (54 casos por 100 mil habitantes), Nordeste (45,2) e Centro Oeste (42,8), em contraste com as regiões Sudeste (14,8) e Sul (27,7). No Norte e no Centro Oeste, representa a principal causa entre todos os tipos de câncer, na população geral.[20]

- 22,1% dos nascidos vivos informados em 1996 provieram de mães com menos de 20 anos de idade. Esse percentual foi de 30% na Região Norte, atingindo valores de 30,5% em Rondônia e Tocantins. As regiões Sudeste e Sul apresentaram taxas de 19,6% e 20,6%, respectivamente.[21]

Recursos e cobertura

- No último levantamento realizado no Brasil, em 1992, havia 36,4 leitos hospitalares

para cada 100 mil habitantes.[22] Porém, as taxas observadas nas regiões Norte e Nordeste (22,3 e 30,4 respectivamente) eram bem inferiores às do Sudeste (40,9), Sul (39,8) e Centro Oeste (41,7). Nova pesquisa está sendo concluída pelo IBGE, com dados atualizados disponíveis até o final de 1999.

- O percentual de óbitos informados sem assistência médica atingiu 20,5% em 1997, no total do país. O percentual por grandes regiões variou de 31,7% no Nordeste a 17,0% na região Sul. Os seguintes estados apresentaram uma proporção mais elevada de óbitos sem assistência médica, indicando dificuldade de acesso a serviços médicos: Acre (49,4%), Paraíba (48,3%), Maranhão (46,7%) e Piauí (46,3%). O estado do Rio Grande do Sul (10,3%) e o Distrito Federal (11,3%) apresentaram as melhores taxas.[23]

- A cobertura da população urbana servida por sistemas de abastecimento de água em rede geral alcançou 76,1% em 1997, variando de 61,3% na Região Nordeste a 87,2% na Região Sudeste. Entre os estados, a cobertura variou de 42,8% no Maranhão a 93,0% e 92,3%, respectivamente, em São Paulo e no Distrito Federal.[24]

- A cobertura com serviços adequados de esgotamento sanitário (ligação em rede ou fossa séptica) alcançou no país a média de 60,0% em 1997, variando de 33,6% na Região Nordeste a 80,9% na Região Sudeste. Entre os estados, as piores coberturas encontram-se no Amapá (12,6%) e em Tocantins (14,0%), e a melhor no Distrito Federal (95,6%).

- A cobertura por coleta regular de lixo foi de 74,0% na média nacional em 1997, variando de 61,8% na Região Norte a 85,8% na Região Sul. Destacam-se com maiores coberturas o

[19] Brasil, Ministério da Saúde, CENEPI. Incidência de doenças transmissíveis. Em: *Rede Interagencial de Informações para a Saúde (RIPSA). Indicadores e dados básicos Brasil, 1998*. Brasília: Ministério da Saúde, CENEPI; 1999.

[20] Brasil, Ministério da Saúde, INCa. Incidência de neoplasias malignas. Em: *Rede Interagencial de Informações para a Saúde (RIPSA). Indicadores e dados básicos Brasil, 1998*. Brasília: Ministério da Saúde, INCa; 1999.

[21] Brasil, Ministério da Saúde, CENEPI. Percentual de nascidos vivos segundo idade das mães. Em: Rede Interagencial de Informações para a Saúde. *Indicadores e dados básicos Brasil, 1997*. Brasília: Ministério da Saúde, CENEPI.; 1998.

[22] Fundação IBGE. Pesquisa de asistência médico-sanitária. Em: *Rede Interagencial de Informações para a Saúde (RIPSA). Indicadores e dados básicos Brasil, 1998*. Brasília: IBGE; 1999.

[23] Brasil, Ministério da Saúde, CENEPI. Proporção de óbitos sem assistência médica. Em: *Rede Interagencial de Informações para a Saúde (RIPSA). Indicadores e dados básicos Brasil, 1997*. Brasília: Ministério da Saúde, CENEPI; 1998.

[24] Fundação IBGE. Indicadores de saneamento básico. Em: *Rede Interagencial de Informações para a Saúde (RIPSA). Indicadores e dados básicos Brasil, 1998*. Brasília: IBGE; 1999.

Distrito Federal (95,5%) e São Paulo (94,4%) e, no outro extremo, o Maranhão (23,4%).

Financiamento/alocação

(a) Gasto federal/estadual/municipal com saúde em relação ao gasto total; (b) alocação de recursos em saneamento básico; (c) gasto com saúde em relação ao PIB; (d) alocação PAB; (e) financiamento do setor. Para os indicadores sugeridos, os dados ainda não estão disponíveis por grandes regiões e estados.

PRIORIDADES E POSSIBILIDADES PARA A COOPERAÇÃO DA OPAS

A Representação da OPAS vem desenvolvendo, em ação conjunta com o Ministério da Saúde e com apoio da Oficina Central, o projeto *Rede Interagencial de Informações para a Saúde — RIPSA*, que visa a disponibilizar um conjunto de indicadores básicos selecionados, preparar informes de situação conjunturais e prospectivos, e reunir bases documentais aplicadas. O sistema está direcionado para a análise de aspectos relevantes para a estruturação e avaliação de políticas e ações públicas de interesse para a saúde, assim como para acompanhar as tendências dos problemas que a OPAS e os governos membros têm como competência manejar. Nos próximos anos, devem desenvolver-se para consolidar a RIPSA, continuar o processo de aperfeiçoamento de indicadores e dados básicos, validar as bases de dados disponíveis e produzir informes analíticos sobre as condições de saúde.

Ainda no campo da informação, a cooperação deverá voltar-se para desenvolver metodologias para a análise de desigualdades e iniqüidades em saúde, mediante a identificação e acompanhamento de indicadores das condições de vida prevalentes. Para isso, a Representação está promovendo parcerias com entidades nacionais especializadas em pesquisa econômica e social, como o IPEA, a Fundação SEADE-SP e a USP.

A OPAS tem a responsabilidade de cooperar, também, no desenvolvimento de estudos de caso sobre o impacto de medidas de intervenção adotadas para reduzir as desigualdades e iniqüidades em saúde. Essa linha de trabalho envolve o estabelecimento de parcerias com entidades nacionais vocacionadas para a realização de pesquisas aplicadas à análise e avaliação de ações e serviços de saúde.

No campo do controle de doenças e agravos à saúde, busca-se revigorar as ações de cooperação para o enfrentamento de grandes problemas persistentes (malária, dengue, doença de Chagas, cólera, lepra e tuberculose), dar suporte aos esforços nacionais para a eliminação de doenças evitáveis por imunização (sarampo e tétano neonatal), e apoiar ações voltadas ao controle de problemas emergentes (aids, entre outros) que requerem iniciativas no campo do desenvolvimento científico e tecnológico.

As ações relativas ao item anterior devem estar balizadas no aprimoramento do sistema de vigilância epidemiológica/vigilância da saúde pública, de forma a proporcionar informação epidemiológica oportuna e base metodológica para o desenho e implementação de medidas de prevenção e controle de doenças, assim como de promoção da saúde. Cumpre à OPAS relevante papel de apoio às iniciativas nacionais nessa área.

Outro ponto focal importante da cooperação refere-se à promoção de programa de vigilância da qualidade de insumos para a saúde, em especial aqueles incluídos nas competências de fundos rotativos administrados pela OPAS. Destacam-se como insumos principais: vacinas e soros, sangue e hemoderivados, medicamentos estratégicos, dispositivos de diagnóstico e produtos destinados ao controle vetorial.

Cabe ainda à OPAS promover o debate sobre o modelo de atenção à saúde e de organização de serviços, no contexto dos marcos referenciais de desenvolvimento do sistema de saúde brasileiro, no sentido de contribuir para o seu contínuo aperfeiçoamento.

EQUIDAD EN MATERIA DE SALUD Y OPORTUNIDAD DE VIDA EN VENEZUELA Y COLOMBIA

Hernán Málaga,[1] Marisela Perdomo,[2] Ángela González[3] y Helena Restrepo[3]

Se presentan en este trabajo los resultados de dos estudios llevados a cabo en Colombia y Venezuela con objeto de analizar las inequidades en salud, en particular en materia de acceso a los servicios de salud y a servicios de salud de igual calidad, y proponer una estrategia de justicia social y de reforma del sector encaminada a corregirlas.

En Venezuela, el estudio se realizó en 1992, sobre la base de datos del censo de 1981 relativos a 707 parroquias con una población de 15 millones de personas (1). El estudio sobre Colombia, llevado a cabo en 1998, se basó en el censo de 1993, que estimó una población de 38 millones de personas (2). El análisis de las inequidades tomó en cuenta las divisiones políticas y el porcentaje de población con necesidades básicas insatisfechas (NBI) en cada unidad geográfica poblacional, agrupadas en Venezuela y Colombia en 10 y 4 estratos socioeconómicos respectivamente.

En Venezuela, 38% de las parroquias pertenecen a estratos con un índice de NBI de 70% a 100%, frente a 23% de los municipios de Colombia. El 8% de los municipios de Colombia presentan un índice de NBI inferior a 30%, frente a 10% de las parroquias de Venezuela. El 10% de la población venezolana vive en parroquias con un índice de NBI de 70% a 100% , frente a 12% de la población colombiana. El 30% de la población venezolana vive en zonas mayormente desarrolladas, frente a 49% de la población colombiana.

En Colombia, el hacinamiento es más frecuente en los municipios con un índice de NBI superior a 70%. En las zonas rurales, los servicios de recolección de basura son prácticamente nulos. La educación presenta una correlación con el desarrollo; la instrucción secundaria y superior tiene una correlación positiva, y el analfabetismo, negativa.

EL MODELO RURAL

Al analizar la mortalidad por estratos socioeconómicos, se observa que en Venezuela el porcentaje correspondiente a la mortalidad por enfermedades transmisibles varía entre 8% y 26%; la mortalidad infantil presenta valores que oscilan entre 10 por 1.000 nacidos vivos y 30 por 1.000 nacidos vivos, y la mortalidad de niños de 1 a 4 años varía de 0,25 a 2,5 por 1.000. El 80% de los casos de tétanos

[1] Representante de OPS/OMS en Colombia.
[2] FUNDEPI, Venezuela.
[3] Instituto Nacional de Salud, Colombia.

neonatal se presenta en comunidades con un índice de NBI superior a 70%.

En Colombia, el porcentaje de enfermedades transmisibles oscila solo de 8% a 10% entre los estratos que presentan menos de 30% de población con NBI y los que tienen más de 70%, pero la proporción de defunciones por diarrea varía de menos de 1% a 2,5%. La escasa correlación probablemente se explique por el hecho de que el porcentaje de defunciones en instituciones de salud varía de 25% a 50%, y el de defunciones sin certificación médica oscila de menos de 1% a más de 28% en los municipios con más de 70% de población con NBI. Hay igualmente una correlación entre el desarrollo y el diagnóstico inexacto de la causa de muerte que oscila entre 1% y 18%, debido sobre todo a que el subregistro de dicha causa se estima en 86% en el estrato más pobre frente a solo 16% en los estratos más desarrollados (3).

EL MODELO URBANO

En Colombia y Venezuela, la mayoría de los municipios o parroquias con altos índices de NBI presentan una elevada proporción de población rural. La búsqueda de mejores oportunidades explica en parte el rápido crecimiento poblacional en las grandes ciudades de ambos países; pero las personas que emigran encuentran deficiencias en lo concerniente a la vivienda, el saneamiento ambiental, el suministro de agua, tanto en cantidad como en calidad, y los servicios de alcantarillado y recolección de basura. Se reproduce así el panorama nacional, con enfermedades relacionadas con la pobreza, como concluye un estudio efectuado en Barquisimeto, Venezuela (4), según el cual la mortalidad infantil varía del 10 por 1.000 nacidos vivos a más de 30 por 1.000 en los barrios más carenciados. De acuerdo con este estudio, el bajo peso al nacer se relaciona con las condiciones de vida, como lo demuestra el hecho de que la mayor cantidad de niños con menos de 2,5 kg de peso nacen en barrios con un índice de NBI superior a 90%. Otros estudios realiza-

dos en Venezuela indican que la talla de los niños que pertenecen a estratos ubicados en los extremos varía de 1,15 m a 1,22 m a los 7 años de edad. Méndez Castellanos señala que esto se traduce en 20 años de diferencia en cuanto al desarrollo biológico entre ambos estratos. Otros datos indican que en Caracas la diferencia entre estratos socioeconómicos en cuanto a la esperanza de vida al nacer varía de 64 a 74 años de edad (5).

En las grandes ciudades también se advierte una correlación entre el desarrollo y las enfermedades cardiovasculares y el cáncer. En Venezuela, la mortalidad por enfermedades cardiovasculares varía entre 35% en las ciudades más grandes y 12% en las más pequeñas. Las neoplasias presentan el mismo cuadro, y si se estudia el cáncer del cuello del útero se puede ver que gran parte del problema radica en las condiciones de pobreza estructural (6). Los mismos resultados se dan en Colombia, donde se advierte una correlación entre el infarto del miocardio y el desarrollo.

En ambos países, la inestabilidad social favorece las enfermedades de transmisión sexual, así como el incremento de los problemas de alcoholismo, drogadicción, crímenes y violencia. En Venezuela los accidentes de vehículos de motor, resultantes de actos de negligencia y violencia, representan 25% del total de años potenciales de vida perdidos, y su prevalencia es mayor en las ciudades con un índice menor de NBI (7). En Colombia los homicidios tienen una correlación con el desarrollo, y en las grandes ciudades se puede observar que los estratos más pobres acusan mayor cantidad de muertes (8).

CONCLUSIÓN

En Colombia y Venezuela, las prioridades sanitarias nacionales declaradas son aumentar la equidad en salud y asegurar el acceso a servicios de salud y a servicios de salud de igual calidad. En el primer caso, la solución es una estrategia de justicia social, y en el segundo, de justicia sanitaria.

ESTRATEGIA DE MUNICIPIOS SALUDABLES

Para impulsar la estrategia de justicia social se ha puesto en marcha el proyecto de municipios saludables (9), en el que la atención primaria de salud busca resolver los problemas sanitarios esenciales en el ámbito local. Esto se ve favorecido por el proceso de descentralización en ambos países y la transferencia de competencias en salud a los municipios. Se privilegia la promoción de la salud y las acciones preventivas, y se ratifica el derecho de todos los habitantes a la salud y a la universalidad de la cobertura, combatiendo las desigualdades sociales y promoviendo la participación ciudadana. La función de liderazgo la ejerce el alcalde, que es quien convoca a todos los sectores de la sociedad. Mediante esta estrategia, y como parte de la misión de salud pública, se busca asegurar las condiciones para el desarrollo de una vida saludable (10). Las principales líneas de acción son la formulación de políticas públicas saludables, la creación de ambientes sanos, el fortalecimiento de la acción comunitaria, la reorientación de los servicios, y el desarrollo de habilidades personales para lograr cambios en el modo de vida (9) y las oportunidades de vida (11).

Un buen ejemplo de políticas públicas saludables es la prohibición del uso de la pólvora en la época de Navidad y Año Nuevo en Bogotá, Colombia, medida que ha logrado reducir la cantidad de niños quemados de 200 a menos de 60 (12). También se ha implantado una política de restricción de la portación de armas, que permitió la disminución de los homicidios con armas de fuego (13). Sobre la base de esta experiencia, una reciente decisión del Presidente de la República impulsa la implantación de esta política en 59 ciudades del país.

Para analizar los problemas de salud hemos recurrido al modelo de Lalonde (14), que facilita el desarrollo de políticas de salud. El control del embarazo en la adolescencia constituye un ejemplo de la aplicación de este modelo. Por ejemplo, tomando en cuenta que el embarazo, que se correlaciona en forma inversa con el desarrollo, es más prevalente en jovencitas que inician su actividad sexual a temprana edad, la intervención modifica el ámbito biológico, el modo de vida. En este sentido, el hecho de estar ocioso explica gran parte del problema y es igualmente relevante el hecho de que la mayor incidencia de embarazo en la adolescencia se observa en muchachas que abandonan los estudios antes de 6 años. Estas variables, junto con algunas respuestas limitadas por parte de los servicios de salud, explican el problema y crean posibilidades de intervención (15).

Con objeto de intervenir ante un problema hemos utilizado el método del marco lógico para diseñar proyectos. Por medio de esta metodología, en Venezuela se estableció un banco con 256 proyectos en 33 de los 64 municipios que están aplicando la estrategia: 36% de los proyectos pertenecen a la esfera de saneamiento básico, 24% a prevención y promoción, 11% a educación, 10% a empleo, y 19% a desarrollo de servicios públicos, incluidos los servicios de salud (16). La ejecución de estos proyectos y programas en el Municipio de Versalles, Colombia, ha afianzado la democracia, favoreciendo la plena participación de la comunidad, ya que es esta la que elabora el plan local de desarrollo. Un efecto indirecto de esta estrategia ha sido la disminución de los homicidios.

REFORMA DEL SISTEMA DE SALUD

Para superar el problema de falta de equidad en el acceso a los servicios de salud, Colombia ha implementado la Ley 100, pero como resultado de los primeros tres años de aplicación, y en un contexto regido por el libre mercado, se han ampliado las brechas, porque las ciudades más grandes recibieron más dinero del régimen subsidiado, mientras que los departamentos más pobres tienen menos población afiliada al sistema de seguridad social. A su vez, esto ha incrementado la inequidad en la cobertura de inmunizaciones debido a la diferencia en el desarrollo de los servicios locales de salud, y así han caído las coberturas de vacunación contra la poliomielitis en todos los departamentos. Este descenso ha sido mayor en los departamentos con elevados índices de NBI (17).

El Plan Nacional de Desarrollo para los años 1999–2000 prevé el incremento de cupos en la cobertura del régimen subsidiado. Este incremento se hará teniendo en cuenta los niveles de NBI y de menor cobertura sanitaria de los diferentes municipios, con miras a corregir el desequilibrio existente entre las diferentes regiones del país. El nivel nacional, por conducto del Fondo de Solidaridad y Garantía (FOSYGA), destinará más recursos para los municipios con mayores porcentajes de población con NBI y menor cobertura, a fin de cumplir con el *principio de equidad y obligatoriedad* que establece la Ley 100 de 1993.

ASPECTOS RELACIONADOS CON LA COOPERACIÓN TÉCNICA

Los principales aspectos relacionados con la cooperación técnica que se ha decidido fortalecer o desarrollar con objeto de aumentar la equidad en salud y el acceso y utilización de los servicios de atención de salud son:

- Focalizar la cooperación técnica en los departamentos y municipios más pobres del país.
- Incluir entre los compromisos de consultores y profesionales nacionales objetivos de disminución de inequidades.
- Desarrollar un sistema de información municipal que comprenda datos de determinantes sociales y ambientales de problemas en salud y promueva el trabajo intersectorial.
- Fomentar la cooperación horizontal mediante la Red Colombiana de Municipios Saludables por la Paz.
- Promover el respeto universal a los derechos humanos, afianzando los procesos de paz y propiciando el incremento del acceso a servicios de salud y educación en las zonas excluidas, por ejemplo mediante pro-

puesta de asignación de recursos del régimen subsidiado a departamentos y municipios con mayores porcentajes de NBI y menos afiliados al sistema de seguridad social, rearticulación de los sistemas locales de salud, abastecimiento universal de agua potable por regímenes de condominio y tecnologías apropiadas, etcétera.

- Reducir las inequidades individuales y sociales por medio de intervenciones preventivas y de promoción de la salud, incluida la capacitación de nuevos actores: alcaldes, secretarios municipales de salud, gerentes de Entidades Promotoras de la Salud (EPS) y de Administradoras del Régimen Subsidiado (ARS), y directores de Instituciones Prestadoras de Servicios de Salud (IPS). Por ejemplo: disminuir la relación entre pobreza estructural y coberturas de inmunización, introducir el enfoque de Atención Integrada a las Enfermedades Prevalentes de la Infancia (AIEPI) en el Plan Obligatorio de Salud (POS), municipios saludables por la paz en los municipios excluidos, CARMEN en grandes ciudades, programas de control de malaria, tuberculosis y lepra en poblaciones vulnerables, etc.
- Asesorar la elaboración de planes de desarrollo de recursos humanos en los niveles departamentales con participación de los nuevos actores.
- Construir un banco de proyectos municipales y propiciar el liderazgo de la Primera Dama, con el propósito de buscar financiamiento para intervenciones locales en municipios y comunidades excluidas.
- El incremento del desplazamiento de población a causa de la violencia ha incrementado las inequidades en el acceso a los servicios de salud. Por ley, la respuesta del Gobierno a esta población sobrepasa la oferta existente en el POS del régimen subsidiado, y se ha creado así un régimen paralelo, por lo que debe propiciarse la elaboración de un modelo cuya aplicación ayude a resolver este grave problema.
- Fomentar la cooperación técnica entre países, sobre todo en las fronteras, con el pro-

pósito de disminuir inequidades en salud, e intercambiar experiencias de estrategias de reforma que hayan ayudado a disminuir las diferencias.

* Divulgar resultados de intervenciones locales, departamentales y nacionales, que reduzcan las inequidades.

REFERENCIAS

1. Universidad Central de Venezuela, Ministerio de Sanidad y Asistencia Social. Perfiles de mortalidad según condiciones de vida: experiencia en Venezuela. *Boletín Epidemiológico* 1993;14(3):11–14.

2. Departamento Autónomo Nacional de Estadística, Ministerio de Salud, Organización Panamericana de la Salud. Condiciones de vida y salud en Colombia. Informe Preliminar. Santa Fe de Bogotá, 1998.

3. Departamento Autónomo Nacional de Estadística, Organización Panamericana de la Salud. Mortalidad según condiciones de vida en Colombia. Jornada Colombiana de Epidemiología, Santa Fe de Bogotá, 1998.

4. Ludewig C, Finizola B, B Gil M, Rivera E, Ugel E, Zeeman P. Propuesta para el análisis de la situación según condiciones de vida de la población para el apoyo a la gestión en niveles locales. IV Reunión Científica Nacional de Epidemiología, San Cristóbal, Venezuela, 1994.

5. Méndez Castellanos H, Paez J. Las circunstancias de enfermarse y morir en Caracas. Estudio sobre mortalidad diferencial en el área metropolitana de Caracas. *Archivos Venezolanos de Puericultura y Pediatría* 1998;61(1):16–26.

6. Venezuela, Ministerio de Sanidad y Asistencia Social, Dirección de Oncología. Epidemiología y la prevención del cáncer uterino. Caracas: Ministerio de Sanidad y Asistencia Social; 1991. (Informe fotocopiado).

7. Venezuela, Ministerio de Sanidad y Asistencia Social. *Políticas de salud en Venezuela*. Caracas: Editorial Gráficas, Chemar; 1992.

8. Guerrero R. La violencia como problema de salud pública en la Región de las Américas. El caso Colombia. En: Memorias de la Conferencia Prevención de la violencia: una oportunidad para los medios de comunicación. 1998. pp. 41–49.

9. Organización Panamericana de la Salud. *Municipios saludables: una estrategia de promoción de la salud en la Organización Panamericana de la Salud en el contexto local*. Washington, DC: OPS; 1992.

10. Mann E. Medicine and public health ethics and human rights. *Hasting Center Report* 1997;27(3):6–13.

11. Kadt E, Tasca R. *Promover la equidad, un nuevo enfoque desde el sector salud*. Washington, DC: Organización Panamericana de la Salud; 1993. (Serie Salud en el Desarrollo).

12. Colombia, Instituto Distrital de Cultura y Turismo, Secretaría Distrital de Salud. Impacto de la restricción para venta y uso de pólvora en Santafé de Bogotá. *El Observatorio de Cultura Urbana* 1997;1(3):1–8.

13. Acero H, Martínez H, Suárez GI, Hernández W. Prevención de lesiones de causas externas en Santafé de Bogotá. *Boletín CRNV* 1996;17(Dic):61–62.

14. Lalonde M. El concepto de "campo de la salud": una perspectiva canadiense. En: Organización Panamericana de la Salud. *Promoción de la salud: una antología*. Washington, DC: OPS; 1996. (Publicación Científica 557).

15. Costagliola A. Factores de riesgo del embarazo precoz en el Municipio Zamora del Estado Falcón, Venezuela [tesis de grado]. Caracas: Universidad Central de Venezuela; 1995.

16. Mandl J, Toba M, eds. Tomo II: Red Venezolana de Municipios hacia la Salud. En: *Municipios hacia la salud: la experiencia venezolana*. Caracas: Organización Panamericana de la Salud, Ministerio de Sanidad y Asistencia Social; 1999.

17. Restrepo H, ed. *Experiencias de municipios saludables por la paz, Colombia*. Santa Fe de Bogotá: Trazo Digital Ltda.; 1999.

18. Málaga H.. Perspectivas de la epidemiología en la reforma de la seguridad social. *Revista de Salud Pública* 1999;1(2):128 B,136 pp.

AGUA PARA TODOS EN EL PAÍS DE LA FANTASÍA

Paulo C. Pinto[1]

Al parodiar la Ficción, la *Realidad* muchas veces nos ofrece incontables oportunidades de buscar alternativas. En "la historia interminable",[2] donde la *Fantasía* y la *Creatividad* van adelante y buscan soluciones, la *Nada* intenta dominar el escenario y establece fronteras a la *Imaginación*.

LA MODERNIZACIÓN DEL ESTADO

A consecuencia de las reformas que han tenido lugar en distintos países de América Latina, el Estado ha pasado a ejercer nuevas funciones. En muchos de ellos, el proceso de privatización procuró vender la imagen de ineficiencia del Estado y de profesionalismo de las empresas privadas. En varios casos, las reformas han llevado aparejada la transferencia de la gestión de los servicios al sector privado, dejando en manos del Gobierno ciertas tareas relativas a la política y planificación sectoriales, así como a la regulación y control. En otros, las políticas y acciones de planificación han sido postergadas. Aunque los países han avanzado en distintos grados y direccio-

nes en sus procesos de reforma, la tendencia podría indicar un movimiento común hacia nuevos modelos de gestión que incorporan al sector privado.

En *Fantasía*, la transformación del sector de la salud se ha orientado a redefinir los papeles de sus actores, básicamente el Estado, que asume las funciones de regulación y control, y el sector privado, a cargo de la prestación de los servicios. Con arreglo a este modelo, se han creado entes reguladores encargados de ejercer las funciones mencionadas por medio de dos instrumentos fundamentales: los marcos regulatorios y los contratos de concesión. De acuerdo con la política de la Administración Nacional, una de las primeras empresas públicas privatizadas fue Obras Sanitarias de Fantasía (OSF). Así, se tomó la decisión de concesionar a un consorcio privado (Aguas de Fantasía, AF) la provisión de agua potable y saneamiento en la capital y ciudades vecinas, cuyo ingreso per cápita era el más significativo del país.

La reforma llevada a cabo consistió en el diseño de un nuevo marco institucional que incluyó la separación de las funciones de prestación de las de regulación, así como la creación de un marco regulatorio del servicio. Esta tarea posibilitó la transferencia de OSF al sector privado (AF) y, simultáneamente, el establecimiento del Ente Regulador de Aguas de Fantasía (ERAF). La experiencia de la con-

---

[1] División Salud y Ambiente, Organización Panamericana de la Salud.

[2] El autor alude a Fantasía, el mágico mundo de lo posible creado por Michael Ende en su novela, *La historia interminable* (Madrid, Alfaguara, 1987). [N del E]

cesión de OSF sirvió como punto de partida para la transformación de los servicios en otras zonas del país.

Si bien ha habido importantes adelantos en cuanto a la ampliación y la calidad de los servicios prestados, el modelo puesto en marcha aún no ha generado los mecanismos adecuados para incrementar significativamente el acceso de los sectores carenciados a los servicios. De hecho, las renegociaciones del contrato de concesión han estado signadas por las dificultades manifestadas por las empresas para cumplir sus obligaciones de ampliación.

En este contexto, deben introducirse nuevos mecanismos en el modelo, reorientando las acciones del Estado tendientes a lograr la cobertura universal de los servicios, mediante la asignación de una alta prioridad al mejoramiento del acceso a estos por parte de los sectores más pobres de la población.

LA TRANSFORMACIÓN Y LOS SECTORES VULNERABLES

Se necesitan modelos capaces de crear mecanismos adecuados y eficientes que permitan extender los servicios a las zonas marginales, teniendo en cuenta que el operador es una empresa privada. Aunque existen algunos elementos comunes, cuando la prestación está a cargo del Estado, este puede fijar las metas de ampliación de los servicios, con lo cual desaparecen los problemas de incentivos inadecuados.

En los últimos tiempos, se ha difundido mucho el concepto de desarrollo sostenible, entendiéndose por tal el desarrollo que permite alcanzar el bienestar de las generaciones actuales sin comprometer el desarrollo de las generaciones futuras. Últimamente, el concepto ha cobrado gran relevancia, y el control de la contaminación se está tornando prioritario para muchas naciones.

Sin embargo, existe controversia en torno al concepto de desarrollo sostenible. Por ejemplo, la Comisión Mundial sobre el Medio Ambiente y el Desarrollo (Comisión Brundtland) condiciona el desarrollo sostenible en América Latina a la posibilidad de encontrar nuevos esquemas para satisfacer las necesidades básicas de la población, en especial de los sectores de bajos recursos que habitan zonas urbanas. La Comisión mencionada profundiza el concepto, planteando un "desarrollo humano sostenible" basado en la urgente erradicación de la pobreza y la solución de los problemas ambientales en las zonas urbanas marginales.

Esta relación entre la disminución de la pobreza y el mejoramiento ambiental también ha sido planteada por instituciones internacionales, tales como la OPS/OMS, el Banco Mundial y el Banco Interamericano de Desarrollo, que han privilegiado el tema de la pobreza en la agenda sanitaria y ambiental de la Región.

La temática del desarrollo sostenible y las oportunidades de alcanzarlo aparece claramente en las zonas urbanas de países en desarrollo. Por lo común, los sectores más perjudicados son los de menores recursos, que sufren en forma directa los efectos de la contaminación y tienen menos posibilidades de acceder a servicios básicos, tales como agua potable y saneamiento. En consecuencia, una vez afectados por la degradación ambiental, no cuentan con los medios para solucionar los problemas ocasionados.

En el ámbito de la concesión de OSF, los principales problemas sanitarios y ambientales están relacionados con los recursos hídricos y los servicios de saneamiento: elevados tenores de contaminación orgánica y tóxica de acuíferos subterráneos, ríos y arroyos (en algunas épocas del año se supera la carga contaminante de los líquidos cloacales); escasa cobertura de servicios, en especial servicios sanitarios; amplios sectores de la población con necesidades básicas insatisfechas.

Estos problemas se han agudizado tanto que los factores de localización que habían sido atractivos para la población —acuíferos subterráneos accesibles y de óptima calidad para el consumo humano, características de absorción de los suelos, aptos para la construcción de pozos y cámaras sépticas, presencia de ríos y arroyos capaces de actuar como cuerpos receptores de efluentes cloacales—, hoy en día se tornan circunstancias negativas, debido a la degradación de sus condiciones naturales y el alto grado de contaminación que presentan, así como a las bajas coberturas de los servicios de saneamiento básico.

Es sabido que los inconvenientes que sufren estas zonas se deben más al crecimiento rápido de las ciudades —que sobrepasa la capacidad de los gobiernos de planificar, financiar y construir nueva infraestructura—, que a su tamaño. A ello se suman las dificultades para mantener la infraestructura existente.

La problemática que afecta a esta área no es privativa de Fantasía. La contaminación del aire, el suelo y el agua en varias ciudades de las Américas ha alcanzado niveles críticos. Como ya se señaló, la mayor incidencia de la contaminación es en la población de bajos recursos, y estos sectores han reconocido que la contaminación constituye uno de sus problemas más importantes. En encuestas realizadas en Fantasía se comprobó que los sectores de bajos recursos estaban dispuestos a pagar importantes sumas (en relación con sus ingresos) a cambio del mejoramiento de las condiciones ambientales de la zona y el acceso a los servicios básicos.

Sin duda, las políticas de ampliación de los servicios de agua potable y saneamiento, y las inversiones en mejoras ambientales en torno a estos servicios, están estrechamente relacionadas con el concepto de desarrollo sostenible, que es más abarcativo que la correspondencia tradicional entre el acceso a los servicios y la salud. En cualquier caso, resulta claro que se requiere una intervención del Estado para establecer las políticas correspondientes. Cuando la prestación de los servicios ha sido concesionada a una empresa privada, es necesario establecer los mecanismos e incentivos adecuados.

EL SISTEMA REGULADOR DE FANTASÍA

La regulación es una función indelegable del Estado, mediante la cual este puede corregir comportamientos monopólicos a partir del establecimiento de normas que orientan o restrinjen decisiones empresarias públicas o privadas.

El desarrollo de los procesos de reforma sectorial en Fantasía ha provocado cambios en los modelos de gestión de los servicios de saneamiento, pues se han puesto en práctica objetivos empresariales e incentivos a la eficiencia susceptibles de crear conflictos de interés entre los prestadores y los usuarios en cuestiones relacionadas con el equilibrio económico-financiero, los niveles de inversión, la calidad de los servicios prestados, o las tarifas. Debido a la posición dominante de los prestadores, los usuarios y la comunidad en su conjunto cuentan con recursos limitados para su protección y defensa.

En este contexto, la regulación de los servicios se concentra en reducir el riesgo de estos conflictos y los comportamientos abusivos resultantes de las posiciones monopólicas. Los sistemas de regulación deben aplicar normas que privilegien en forma distinta los tres aspectos principales del servicio público en los que pueden originarse comportamientos perjudiciales en relación con el costo, la calidad o la cantidad. Es claro que la aplicación de una norma que exige costos mínimos a los usuarios puede inducir niveles inadecuados de calidad del servicio, así como establecer parámetros exigentes en términos de calidad puede inducir altos costos y tarifas.

LA EVOLUCIÓN DE LOS SERVICIOS EN FANTASÍA

El contrato de concesión en Fantasía estableció una serie de objetivos relacionados con la mejora de la calidad de los servicios, el incremento de las coberturas de agua potable y saneamiento, y la concreción de determinadas inversiones. Al comparar la situación del comienzo de la concesión con la correspondiente a la finalización del primer quinquenio, de manera sintética puede señalarse lo siguiente:

- Los servicios mejoraron significativamente, tanto en relación a la calidad del agua distribuida como a algunos parámetros físicos, a saber: presión del agua; control de las descargas cloacales; tratamiento de las aguas residuales, y otros;
- La población con servicio de agua potable aumentó un 13%, y la incorporada al sistema de alcantarillado cloacal, 6%. Aunque se trató de aumentos importantes, no se alcanzaron las metas establecidas en el contrato de concesión.

Una de las cuestiones críticas relacionadas con la ampliación de los servicios fue el fracaso del denominado "cargo de infraestructura", una contribución que los nuevos usuarios debían pagar a la empresa concesionaria en concepto de acceso a los servicios (fijado en $ 500 y $ 1000, por conexión de agua y alcantarillado, respectivamente). Cuando la ampliación alcanzó a los sectores de bajos recursos, surgieron problemas de cobro de la contribución mencionada, en razón de los costos elevados, que estos sectores no estaban en condiciones de cubrir. Esto llevó a una renegociación del contrato entre el Estado y la empresa concesionaria, AF, que finalizó con la promulgación de un decreto en el que se estableció que la ampliación de los servicios debía financiarse mediante el denominado cargo al servicio universal ($ 1,0 por servicio, por mes), que los usuarios existentes pagarían como parte de su tarifa.

Sin embargo, por diferentes razones, este esquema de subsidios cruzados para financiar la ampliación de los servicios también fue dejado de lado, proponiéndose actualmente un sistema de financiamiento con la participación de otros actores interesados en la solución. Consiste en el establecimiento de convenios entre el municipio y los habitantes de la zona a la que se va a extender el servicio, de acuerdo con los cuales este selecciona una empresa constructora que ejecuta las obras y las transfiere al concesionario privado y, una vez habilitado el servicio, los usuarios pagan en cuotas las inversiones correspondientes. La ventaja aparente de este sistema radica en que aparecen nuevas fuentes de recursos, ajenos a los que puede generar la empresa concesionaria, y el problema que podría surgir es, nuevamente, el de las dificultades de los sectores de bajos recursos para pagar las cuotas correspondientes.

CUESTIONES PARA RESPONDER EN LA AMPLIACIÓN DE LOS SERVICIOS A LAS ZONAS MARGINADAS

La situación descripta, que ha enfrentado la concesión de Fantasía, coincide con la de otras ciudades de la Región, con modelos de prestación de servicios, tanto públicos como privados. Surgen, entonces, las siguientes preguntas, para los casos en que los servicios han sido dados en concesión a una empresa privada:

- ¿Cómo generar recursos para la ampliación de los servicios en las zonas marginales?
- ¿Debe el Estado intervenir en el financiamiento cuando el prestador es una empresa privada?
- ¿Es viable que las obras de ampliación las ejecute el Estado y luego las transfiera a la empresa concesionaria para su explotación?
- ¿Que mecanismo es más eficiente: los subsidios cruzados o los subsidios directos?
- ¿Cuáles deben ser los incentivos y obligaciones que deben establecerse, de manera que las empresas ejecuten la ampliación de los servicios de acuerdo con las metas establecidas?
- ¿Cómo puede organizarse la comunidad? (esquemas de aporte de materiales y mano de obra)
- ¿Cuáles son las tecnologías apropiadas?
- ¿Pueden establecerse niveles de servicio diferenciados?
- ¿Cuáles deben ser los arreglos institucionales?
- ¿Cuáles son las funciones del Estado (en sus diferentes niveles), del ente regulador, de la empresa privada, de las organizaciones no gubernamentales y de la comunidad organizada.

Ética, Equidad y Práctica en las Instituciones de Salud

Fernando Lolas Stepke[1]

PREÁMBULO

El Director de la Oficina Sanitaria Panamericana (Organización Panamericana de la Salud), George A. O. Alleyne, ha pensado que
algunas de mis reflexiones previamente pu-
blicadas podrían resultar de interés para este
público.[2] Hoy nos congrega una dimensión
valórica del trabajo de la Organización que requiere tiempo y reflexión para ser correcta-
mente aprehendida. En realidad, el tema de
la equidad es una vía de entrada al universo
conceptual y moral de los supuestos que ani-
man dicho trabajo.

NADA HAY MÁS PRÁCTICO QUE UNA BUENA TEORÍA

Para caracterizar el saber teórico, decía Ortega y Gasset que era aquella forma de saber

que, tomando distancia de las solicitaciones
de lo inmediato, contempla la totalidad de las
capacidades del intelecto y encuentra el significado en esa contemplación. No en vano la
voz *teoría* recuerda al teatro, aquel sitio privilegiado en que el mundo y la gente se ofrecen
como espectáculo a la mirada.

Por cierto, en las disciplinas científico-na-
turales tiene la voz teoría la acepción más
modesta de compacto resumen de observaciones que permite predicción y anticipación. Sin
embargo, es la noción intuitiva de teoría como
aprehensión de totalidades significativas la
que quisiera destacar en esta ocasión.

Gracias al saber teórico, y al tipo de praxis
reflexiva que él permite, podemos *des-cubrir* lo
obvio, revelar las implícitas certidumbres que
impregnan nuestras prácticas habituales y los
axiomas de nuestro quehacer y, cuando es exi-
toso el esfuerzo, deshacer las inercias del hábito y poner en entredicho lo que parece simple.
Gracias a la pupila teórica podemos "desen-
mascarar lo real", mostrarlo en la infinita variedad de sus circunstanciales apariencias y
reforzar con ello la eficacia de nuestros actos.

Por eso es tan valioso, y por valioso escaso,
el privilegio de tomar distancia de las incita-
ciones de lo inmediato y retirarse a la reflexión.
Este interludio, que es retiro y trabajo teórico,
es un bien mayor. Permite esa *cronofilia* bené-
fica del ocio regio, que ama al tiempo y per-

---

[1] Director del Programa Regional de Bioética, Organización Panamericana de la Salud. El texto reconstruye la conferencia pronunciada el 28 de octubre de 1999 en la reunión
de gerentes de la OPS que se realizó en Washington, D.C.
Las afirmaciones son de la exclusiva responsabilidad del autor y no suponen reconocimiento ni respaldo institucional.

[2] Algunos de los temas y argumentos se encuentran,
entre otros, en los libros: *Notas al margen*, Editorial Cuatro Vientos, Santiago de Chile, 1985, *Proposiciones para una
teoría de la medicina*, Editorial Universitaria, Santiago de
Chile, 1992, *Ensayos sobre ciencia y sociedad*, Estudios Sigma,
Buenos Aires, 1995, *Más allá del cuerpo*, Editorial Andrés
Bello, Santiago de Chile, 1997.

mite superar la *cronofobia* de la acción urgente, en que el apremio no admite opciones. Quienes laboran en el campo de la salud encuentran a menudo que carecen de tiempo y de quietud para rescatar la misteriosa energía de lo nuevo y revitalizar las fuentes del entusiasmo. Lo importante no es siempre lo más urgente. Y la teoría es importante.

Lo es por varios motivos. Es, primeramente, inevitable. Todo el mundo construye teorías, da ciertas cosas por supuestas, anticipa el desarrollo de los acontecimientos sobre la base de algún modelo o principio. No hay saber enseñable que carezca de teoría, pues para enseñar se precisa un esquema global de aquello que se enseña. Y, finalmente, como ya señalamos, la teoría proporciona los cimientos de toda práctica reglada. Al hacer, agrega el saber y convierte la acción experta en un *saber-hacer*. Este es el fundamento de las profesiones modernas basadas en las tecnociencias y deudoras de su empiria sistemática.

De allí la conclusión: nada hay más práctico que una buena teoría.

LA EXPLICITACIÓN DE LOS CONCEPTOS ÉTICOS ES TAREA DE LA REFLEXIÓN

Particular relieve tiene, en este contexto, que se nos invite a reflexionar sobre filosofía moral. Hoy preferimos para ese viejo menester el término *ética*, que es a la moral lo que la musicología a la música, esto es, su fundamentación racional y su sustrato teórico. No es tanto explicar lo que hacemos en términos de maldad o bondad cuanto explicitar los términos que usamos y dar razón de nuestro comportamiento, lo que constituye lo más esencial del discurso ético contemporáneo. Refraseado como *bioética* en el ámbito de las tecnociencias sobre la vida y la salud es, como toda disciplina, un *discurso*. Esto significa la fusión de hablante y de lengua en formas creativas y novedosas, con una retórica y un interés social, y, sobre todo, con la facultad de *crear los objetos* de los cuales hablar. Una disci-

plina es un discurso que genera aquello de lo que habla, lo construye para la mirada, lo desconstruye para el análisis y lo reconstruye para la acción.

En el caso de la bioética en tanto que discurso, a las acepciones tradicionales de ética como costumbre o hábito, y ética como carácter, ha venido a agregarse, en mi opinión de modo sustantivo, la dimensión dialógica. Bioética es, por ende, un discurso constitutivamente dialógico, una narrativa social que ilumina el imaginario moral de nuestras prácticas y las somete al juicio y a la crítica.

Todas las formas de filosofía moral —o ética en sentido amplio, incluida la mutación bioética— tienen entre sus metas definir y explicitar dos conceptos: el de lo bueno y el de lo justo. Al hacerlo, derivan hacia principios universales, generales y públicos, que señalan las formas usuales de fundamentar y aplicar las nociones esenciales.

Lo bueno puede ser predicado con independencia de lo justo. Definido en primer término, aparece lo justo como el modo adecuado de lograr lo bueno, y todas las doctrinas teleológicas de la moral comparten ese carácter. Lo bueno puede ser definido en relación a la perfección o virtud (perfeccionismo), en relación al placer (hedonismo), en relación a la felicidad (eudemonismo), por citar algunos de una larga lista de ejemplos.

Otros autores, de persuasiones diferentes, sugieren una definición procesal y contractual de la justicia. Esto significa, por una parte, renunciar a compartir una narrativa fundante que nos vinculara a todos en la convicción y certidumbre de lo bueno y, por ende, digno de ser buscado. Las sociedades contemporáneas son mosaicos de pluralidades. *Pluralismo moral* que nos convierte, en el decir de Tristram Engelhardt, en "extraños morales". Pero también, y no tan independiente del primero, *pluralismo epistémico*, que hace diferente el saber según el contexto y el grupo social que lo atesora y perfecciona.

Pienso que la popularidad de la teoría de la justicia de John Rawls se debe, aparte de su intrínseca geometría y articulación, a responder a este carácter formal —procedimental— de la concepción de lo justo y al empleo de la metáfora del "velo de la ignorancia", que Rawls declara esencialmente kantiana.[3] Según esta noción, una sociedad ideal, en su punto de partida, está conformada por seres racionales, desinteresados, libres de odio y envidia, que deciden ponerse de acuerdo sobre los principios de justicia que deberían adoptar. En esa búsqueda, llegan a los famosos dos principios que Rawls enuncia, el de la libertad y el de la diferencia, que en la ficción de esa utopía serán escogidos como los que mejor aseguran la convivencia.

Para abordar el problema de la equidad, las nociones de lo bueno y de lo justo son indispensables y debieran ser explicitadas por todo aquel que desee hacerlo. La esencia de la doctrina de Rawls es que la justicia es, fundamentalmente, equidad. Y equidad significa algo así como imparcialidad y proporcionalidad apropiada en la distribución de los bienes, los honores y los beneficios. No igualdad, sino distribución proporcionada a los merecimientos debidos a cada uno. Se dirá, entonces, de una diferencia que es inequidad cuando es injusta, y puede serlo por ser innecesaria, evitable, involuntaria o atribuible a algún agente. Sobra agregar que las personas y los grupos siempre se caracterizan por sus distinciones y diferencias, y afirman su identidad por medio de ellas. Algunas distinciones no comportan diferencias. Algunas diferencias no llegan a frasearse como distinciones. Pero, de entre las diferencias, las que son injustas por los motivos indicados son llamadas inequidades.

Estas diferencias injustas en los servicios de promoción, protección y recuperación de la salud, estas inequidades, son, sin duda, un excelente motivo para la acción de instituciones de servicio público. El modo en que se aborde su análisis o se promueva su disminución o

remoción, siempre es un tema moral. Lo que importa examinar no es solamente su forma o sus manifestaciones. Interesa también estudiar cómo podrían encararse las acciones en el seno de las distintas sociedades, y qué discurso debe emplearse para convencer a quienes toman decisiones políticas sobre cuáles son los modelos apropiados de intervención.

Sabido es que al respecto se ofrecen varias alternativas. Tal vez la más obvia sea el pensamiento utilitarista, que busca el máximo bien para el mayor número, prestando atención escasa a la distribución de ese bien. Así, por ejemplo, el observar un aumento en el promedio de la esperanza de vida mediante intervenciones apropiadas convencería a un utilitarista sobre la bondad de su acción. Aunque ello pudiera implicar pérdida de otros bienes y aunque fuera inequitativo el beneficio. Por otra parte, aunque se promuevan fines sociales puede existir, soterrado, un pensamiento individualista que, bajo la consigna del igualitarismo, se resigne a una acción que no toma en cuenta las notables disparidades de oportunidad y acceso en materia de educación que padecen numerosas sociedades y grupos en nuestra Región.

El análisis podría extenderse. Sin embargo, el punto es el siguiente: toda reflexión y toda teoría cumplen su propósito si contribuyen a explicitar los supuestos que implícita o explícitamente fundamentan las conductas. Explicitar no consiste solo en explicar: consiste en "abrir" cada concepto del lenguaje común o del técnico, examinar sus resonancias, estudiar sus connotaciones y abrirse a sus infinitas posibilidades en la imaginación social.

DE LAS INSTITUCIONES SOCIALES QUE SATISFACEN DEMANDAS

Las necesidades y los deseos de las personas, cuando son reconocidos y se anhela su satisfacción, pasan a constituirse en *demandas*. Estas son, por tanto, necesidades y deseos que para su satisfacción exigen un esfuerzo deci-

[3] Rawls J. *A Theory of Justice*. Cambridge, Massachusetts: Harvard University Press; 1971. [Versión en español: *Teoría de la justicia*. 2a ed. México: Fondo de Cultura Económica; 1995.]

dido y consciente. Cuestan dinero o tiempo. Quienes resuelven demandas gozan de los reconocimientos de los grupos humanos: prestigio, dinero, poder, amor.

Una *institución social* es un agregado de personas, relaciones entre personas, objetos, conceptos y recursos, que responde a una demanda social. Responder a una demanda significa que hay interés en su existencia, e interés significa relación (Inter-Esse, entre seres) de personas con personas y de personas con cosas. Del estudio de las instituciones se infiere que materializan *sistemas de reglas relacionales* de naturaleza pública, esto es, evidenciable, y que su acción consiste casi siempre en la creación, el perfeccionamiento o la aplicación de una o varias tecnologías.

La voz *tecnología* tiene en este contexto un significado preciso. Significa, como su etimología más auténtica sugiere, logos de la técnica. Esto es, técnica —un hacer—, con un contexto racional que la dota de significado social —un saber—. Decíamos antes: saber-hacer. Las profesiones modernas y el saber experto que valoran hoy las sociedades son amalgamas de saber y de hacer. Ni pura técnica ni pura teoría. Una mezcla. Una proporción adecuada de ambas.

Las instituciones sociales de servicio sirven mediante tecnologías. Por ejemplo, tecnologías *productivas*, que producen bienes (*poiesis*) o procesos sociales (*praxis*). Tecnologías *semióticas*, que trabajan con signos y símbolos, produciéndolos, modificándolos o eliminándolos. Tecnologías *organizacionales*, que se refieren a la constitución y distribución del poder y al establecimiento de jerarquías. Y tecnologías *del sí mismo*, que establecen y modifican identidades.

Sostengo que estas cuatro clases de tecnologías están involucradas en todo tipo de institución social en grados y proporciones diferentes según sus finalidades. Es hasta posible argumentar que una misma institución, a lo largo de su historia, puede cambiar su tecnología dominante y, con ello, su carácter.[4] Lo

esencial no es hacer aquí una taxonomía institucional —puede ello tener inmenso beneficio—, sino destacar que una institución social nace en respuesta a una demanda (necesidad o deseo con precio), materializa un interés de la comunidad (garantía de su existencia), y manipula tecnologías.

INSTITUCIONES SOCIALES Y SU VIRTUD PRIMORDIAL: LA JUSTICIA

Dice John Rawls que la primera virtud de toda institución social es la *justicia*, así como la verdad es la virtud primordial de los sistemas de pensamiento.

Entre las creencias y las normas, en el amplio espacio de la convivencia y del diálogo, las instituciones suelen convertir los ideales en principios prácticos y las ideas en acciones. Una nueva concepción del mundo, por ejemplo, fruto de las instituciones académicas, influye sobre procesos sociales a través de personas que la transforman en inspiración de sus actos. Un valor religioso, que las iglesias transforman en culto y ritual, compite con otros valores para determinar la conducta de los individuos. Y así, en general, puede descubrirse que las instituciones, por obra misma de su existir, manifiestan la textura valórica de la sociedad mayor, y esta puede estudiarse con provecho atendiendo al tipo, variedad y calidad de las instituciones sociales.

Cuando se examina el trabajo de algunas instituciones sociales, suele describírselo en términos tales como "operacionalizar" conceptos y diseñar estrategias de aplicación de conocimientos para intervenir en la marcha de la sociedad. Tal es el caso de las organizaciones vinculadas a la salud y el bienestar. Como la mayoría de ellas basa su eficacia en procesos cognoscitivos y en sus resultados, los examinaremos brevemente en el contexto del trabajo institucional.

---

[4] Cf. Lolas F. Medical praxis: an interface between ethics, politics, and technology. *Social Science and Medicine* 1994;39:1–5. Lolas F. Theoretical medicine: a proposal for reconceptualizing medicine as a science of actions. *The Journal of Medicine and Philosophy* 1996;21:659–670.

INVENCIÓN, INNOVACIÓN, TRANSFORMACIÓN SOCIAL

Los procesos que influyen en la salud y el bienestar pueden englobarse en tres grandes grupos. Por un lado, la *invención*, que siempre lo es de conceptos e ideas. Puede definírsela como la creación de posibilidades de experiencia, como un aumento del "input" potencial de un sistema de creencias y acciones. Un concepto como el de átomo, por ejemplo, es una invención fértil porque permite acomodar muchos hechos perceptivos y de experiencia, o incluso anticipar hechos que no existen aún. La invención siempre es un proceso teórico, un anticipar experiencias posibles. Cuando Ortega y Gasset habla de los conceptos, en realidad piensa en ellos como herramientas para construir mundos. Los conceptos, en tanto invenciones, son "constructos". Son construidos y construyen. La fuerza indiscutible de las tecnologías sanitarias procede de invenciones afortunadas.

El proceso de *innovación* consiste en aumentar el "output" de una determinada construcción conceptual. Es, por ejemplo, el perfeccionamiento de técnicas. Es incrementar el campo de aplicaciones de una teoría. Es, en síntesis, sacar el máximo provecho a lo que ya existe, mejorar en sentido cualitativo y cuantitativo lo que se tiene. La mayor parte de los instrumentos y artefactos que hoy empleamos son perfeccionamientos innovadores de algo que ya existía.

Hay un tercer conjunto de procesos que no se dejan describir en los términos empleados para hablar de innovación e invención. Aunque es posible que, en último análisis, toda *transformación social* dependa de uno de aquellos dos procesos, es preferible —heurísticamente preferible— mantener una designación especial para las mutaciones del alma colectiva que pueden preceder, acompañar o seguir a la invención y la innovación. La conveniencia de separar la transformación social se ejemplifica al considerar que inventos fascinantes, de evidente utilidad, no tuvieron eco en la sociedad de su tiempo, y que, a la inversa, modificaciones del escenario social hicieron imperativa la aparición de ciertos inventos o la innovación de algunas técnicas. Es probable que el sustrato en que acontece la transformación social sea ese magma germinal indiferenciado que los autores franceses han llamado "mentalidad". Una forma especial de existir las comunidades, una modulación del ser humano social que constituye una manifestación peculiar susceptible de cambio, progreso y retroceso. La historia de las mentalidades es la historia de las posibilidades diferentes de habitar el mundo y de dotar de sentido a la información, el conocimiento y las emociones. La transformación de las mentalidades es un proceso que analíticamente podemos independizar de la innovación y la invención.

Estos tres tipos de procesos, invención, innovación y transformación social, pueden concebirse ligados en secuencia lineal. Clásicamente se ha pensado que la invención —la ciencia pura y la investigación fundamental— precede a la innovación, y que esta no es sino su aplicación que produce transformación social al ser generalizada o hecha industria. Pasteur decía: "no existen la ciencia y la técnica, solo la ciencia y las aplicaciones de la ciencia".

Hay varios motivos para dudar de esta secuencia lineal. Aunque no procede discutirlo aquí, baste observar que la innovación produce más innovación, y a veces decide el curso de la invención. La ciencia moderna sería impensable sin tecnologías apropiadas para sus cada vez más exactas preguntas. No toda invención fructifica o es aceptada socialmente, y ello se demuestra con el ejemplo de la energía nuclear aplicada a usos pacíficos, que siendo tecnología apropiada y brillante demostración de ingenio, supone riesgos que algunas sociedades rechazan. Ya hemos mencionado la fascinante hipótesis de que la transformación espiritual de una sociedad, una mutación de su sensibilidad o mentalidad, haga necesario cierto tipo de invención o demande algunas innovaciones específicas.

Por lo tanto, es posible proponer que en lugar de una secuencia nos encontramos con un interminable ciclo de recurrencia entre la invención, la innovación y la transformación social. Cada proceso está determinado y a su vez codetermina los otros. El resultado final quizá no pueda ser retrotraído a una causa única ni anticipado como consecuencia simple de un solo conjunto de procesos.

DEMANDAS ÉTICAS AL TRABAJO INSTITUCIONAL

La mejor manera de anticipar el futuro es inventarlo. Si algo caracteriza la actual demanda de reflexión y de diálogo bioético es la comprobación de que serán efectivos no solamente si reaccionan frente a yerros o excesos sino, y muy especialmente, si los anticipan y previenen. La *actitud proactiva* en filosofía moral puede caracterizarse como el intento por iniciar el ciclo invención-innovación-transformación en el plano de la sensibilidad vital, o al menos considerar esta desde que se piensa en nuevos conocimientos o se realizan innovaciones técnicas. Así, por ejemplo, sabido es que una innovación en medicina crea condiciones problemáticas respecto del acceso a ella. Es obvio que la racionalidad tecnocrática, al hacerse hegemónica, empieza a responder a sus propias exigencias y se libera de compromisos con la demanda que la hizo necesaria. Muchos adelantos llamados médicos son en realidad tecnocráticos y no responden ya a la inicial demanda de atención sanitaria. Piénsese tan solo en la mayor resolución de los aparatos de imaginología que incrementan a veces marginalmente la precisión diagnóstica, pero que la industria hace creer que son fundamentales para la atención correcta. O considérese que, al bajar el "umbral tecnológico de detección de anomalías", muchas condiciones asintomáticas (alto colesterol sanguíneo, presión arterial elevada) se convierten en auténticas "enfermedades" que exigen intervención. Paradójico es, pero real, que muchos perfeccionamientos e innovaciones, aparentemente susceptibles de ser reconstruidos como respuestas a la demanda inicial (atención de salud), en último análisis son inherentes a la dinámica de una institución social distinta, el sistema tecnológico y su correspondiente tecnocracia dominante. La reflexión ética proactiva es hoy día indispensable para anticipar y, ojalá, atenuar la patogenicidad del progreso y la inevitable faz jánica de las tecnociencias: como el dios Jano, sus resultados tienen dos caras y pueden ser deletéreos o benéficos, dependiendo de muchos factores, la demanda entre otros.

Es también un imperativo ético que las instituciones de servicio aclaren los alcances de su acción y *despierten expectativas razonables* sobre su efectividad y eficacia. Articular las demandas significa justamente eso: ser realista en lo que se ofrece y no despertar esperanzas vacías de contenido. Toda institución que construye futuro debe hacerlo con la responsabilidad inherente a su credibilidad y al respeto que inspira. No hay que olvidar que tanto como el resultado de una intervención técnica importa su *significado* social, y este opera en el plano de la sensibilidad vital, de la mentalidad y del espíritu comunitario. Siempre hay un "doble efecto": por un lado, el resultado concreto, por otro, el simbólico. A veces prevalece este último, y una institución que demuestra ser eficaz por cifras interesantes de reducción de morbilidad y mortalidad puede carecer de crédito público por razones que nada tienen que ver con su competencia.

Cada institución de servicio en el campo de la salud, al articular la demanda y definir el ámbito de sus intervenciones define al mismo tiempo la efectividad de su acción posible. Llamo *efectividad* al resultado de la acción óptima en condiciones ideales, es decir, tal y como lo imaginan los planificadores. Como es sabido, se trata de útiles ficciones y nunca se dan integralmente en el mundo real. Cuando hablamos de este, la efectividad se transforma en *eficacia*, es decir, el real resultado en condiciones reales. Obsérvese que la *eficiencia* es el cumplimiento de la eficacia, y es un valor ético tanto como organizacional o administrativo. No se está obligado a realizar el mejor de los mundos posibles, sino a perfeccionar el más concreto de los mundos reales. Nunca la ética ha significado prometer y realizar imposibles.

Hacer transparente la toma de decisiones es un imperativo ético porque la justicia, primer valor de toda institución social, se basa en buena medida en la imparcialidad. La publicidad, aunque el término sea engañosamente trivializante, es una obligación ética que en las instituciones de servicio adquiere importancia en diversos planos. Sin duda en el plano técnico, pues muchas de las acciones de tales instituciones consisten en transformar los datos en informaciones, y estas en conocimiento. Hay aquí un imperativo ético, una verdadera "eticidad" del saber que debe estudiarse y perfeccionarse. El servicio sanitario es tanto una conversión de ideas en acciones cuanto un adaptar estas al cambiante escenario de las demandas humanas. Hablar de equidad requiere tener en cuenta que se trata de un constructo de extrema labilidad, móvil como una veleta, que requiere conciencia vigilante y absoluta transparencia en los conceptos y sus aplicaciones.

Hay en toda institución de servicio que perfecciona sus conceptos y sus técnicas el riesgo propio de las expertocracias, al que ya nos hemos referido diciendo que el sistema tecnológico empieza a responder a su grupo de referencia, la tecnocracia, y olvida su papel mediador del bienestar humano. También las tecnologías "blandas", de la organización y la gerencia, tienen ese riesgo. Embelesados por sus logros, conscientes de su autosuficiencia, los gerentes y administradores pueden fácilmente olvidar el fin último de su trabajo. No es éste perfeccionar sus instrumentos, realizar proezas de eficiencia, lograr excelentes índices de costo/beneficio, sino simplemente, servir al bienestar y la salud. Necesitamos, hoy más que antes, *una reflexión que se concentre en los fines y no solamente en los medios*. Una ética de fines no es necesariamente una ética comprometida con una narrativa exclusiva y excluyente. Los fines no son patrimonio exclusivo de ninguna religión o ideología. Los fines son también materia de consenso social, y, por ende, de diálogo. También, por cierto, de adecuados procedimientos para precisarlos, legítimos en tanto que

voluntariamente formulados y aceptados por toda la comunidad.

Toda la comunidad implica *participación*. En ninguna otra esfera se demuestra mejor la veracidad del aserto "saber es participar" que en la sanitaria. Saber es "tomar parte" en el diálogo social y ser reconocido como poseedor de la capacidad de dialogar. La ética del discurso no es sino el sencillo reconocimiento de que la praxis comunicativa supone agentes morales y epistémicos reconocibles en tanto capaces de diálogo eficaz y no solamente como reflejos o receptores de conocimiento experto. La tradicional verticalidad del discurso profesional y técnico ha sido erosionada por la necesaria *horizontalidad* que demandan las más importantes acciones en salud. Nada saca un gobierno invirtiendo en costosos aparatos si la gente no puede participar en su uso adecuado. La equidad es aquí *equidad de acceso al conocimiento*, con las particularidades de este según el contexto en que se forja y aplica. Está demostrado que la jerga expertocrática, que desdeña o ignora el sentir de las personas a las que dice servir, se esteriliza y aísla, haciéndose al final inútil. El imperativo bioético del diálogo adquiere una máxima prioridad en el diseño del futuro.

Las instituciones sociales que laboran en pro de la salud y del bienestar deben demostrar su eficiencia con *respuestas acordes a demandas razonables*. Ya esta afirmación es compleja, toda vez que lo razonable de una demanda suele ser materia de discrepancias entre los que la experimentan y los que debieran satisfacerla. Lo que "tratamiento adecuado" significa en Manhattan, es distinto en Bucaramanga. El lenguaje de la oferta no siempre concuerda con el de la demanda, y el resultado de esta discrepancia es frustración e insatisfacción de usuarios y proveedores de servicios. Planificar sin actuar no satisface adecuadamente y es imperativo ético demostrar con acciones lo que se predica.

Queda para el final la más crítica, la más importante y definitiva de las exigencias éticas: se resume ella en la *excelencia técnica*. Nada que se haga en forma imperfecta, liviana, descuidada, puede ser moralmente aceptable, así sea inspirado por la intención más beneficiadora que se pueda imaginar, o signifique en realidad un alivio para los que sufren. Como debe leerse el juramento hipocrático es que no puede haber un médico bueno si antes no se es buen médico. La competencia técnica es el primer imperativo ético de todas las profesiones y oficios creados para ayudar a las personas. El compromiso es mantener constante el afán de perfección.

LO PROPIO, LO BUENO, LO JUSTO

En modo alguno agotan las reflexiones precedentes las cuestiones que genera la pregunta por la impronta ética de una institución de servicio. Más bien quedan como provisional incitación a un desarrollo deseable.

Tener espacio para la reflexión y la práctica de la teoría es un privilegio, pero también una obligación. Obliga en realidad a una postura permanentemente crítica de lo que se hace, de sus motivaciones y de sus resultados.

El resumen de este ejercicio es simple y directo. Las acciones han de ser apropiadas, en el sentido de cumplir con las exigencias del buen arte. Lo propio es el primer valor, el valor técnico, lo bien pensado y ejecutado. La *mathesis*.

Lo bien hecho está bien porque cumple con el recto proceder, pero también porque consigue buenos resultados. Entre ellos, hacer bueno al agente que ejecuta la acción, ser su camino y posibilidad de perfección, su *askesis*.

La acción correcta de una institución de servicio y ayuda debe ser además justa. La justicia, primera virtud de toda institución social en tanto que tal, debe extenderse a sus acciones hacia la comunidad. Y justas son las acciones que, si se generalizaran, acrecerían los beneficios, el bienestar y la felicidad del cuerpo social.

Tales son, en suma, las dimensiones del juicio bioético: lo propio, lo bueno y lo justo.[5] Pienso que las demás pueden derivarse de ellas.

---

[5] Cf. Lolas F. *Bioética y antropología médica*. Santiago de Chile: Editorial Mediterráneo; 1999.